"Pain is the most psychological of all topics. We learn here that it has always been a conceptual, methodological, philosophical, and at times troubling challenge for psychology. Kugelmann provides a scholarly, but thoroughly accessible, treatment of pain and our attempts to understand what it teaches about the human condition."

Christopher Eccleston, University of Bath, UK

"Wide-ranging scholarship and keen critical insight are combined with phenomenological research in this outstanding contribution to our understanding of pain. At the same time, Kugelmann reaches beyond intellectual understandings to touch the deeply personal experience of pain. An invaluable resource for both researchers and practitioners interested in this profoundly human topic."

Michael P. Sipiora, Pacifica Graduate Institute, USA

"A fascinating account of different approaches to the study of pain which Kugelmann connects with his own research on narratives of chronic pain. I liked the way he connects our personal experience of pain with our experience of living in a troubled world. As he says: "Pain [. . .] is not private. It connects us with a broken world". A truly original contribution to the literature."

Michael Murray, Keele University, UK

CONSTRUCTING PAIN

Everyone experiences pain, whether it's emotional or physical, chronic or acute. Pain is part of what it means to be human, and so an understanding of how we relate to it as individuals – as well as cultures and societies – is fundamental to who we are.

In this important new book, the first in Routledge's new *Critical Approaches to Health* series, Robert Kugelmann provides an accessible and insightful overview of how the concept of pain has been understood historically, psychologically, and anthropologically. Charting changes in how, after the development of modern painkillers, pain became a problem that could be solved, the book articulates how the possibilities for living with pain have changed over the last two hundred years.

Incorporating research conducted by the author himself, the book provides both a holistic conception of pain and an understanding of what it means to people experiencing it today. Including critical reflections in each chapter, *Constructing Pain* offers a comprehensive and enlightening treatment of an important issue to us all and will be fascinating reading for students and researchers within health psychology, health care, and nursing.

Robert Kugelmann is a professor of psychology at the University of Dallas, USA. He is the author of *Stress* (1992) and *Psychology and Catholicism* (2011), as well as articles on the history of psychology and health psychology.

Critical Approaches to Health

Series Editors: Kerry Chamberlain and Antonia Lyons

The Routledge *Critical Approaches to Health* series aims to present critical interdisciplinary books around psychological, social, and cultural issues related to health. Each volume in the series provides a critical approach to a particular issue or important topic and is of interest and relevance to students and practitioners across the social sciences. The series is produced in association with the International Society of Critical Health Psychology (ISCHP).

Titles in the series

Constructing Pain
Historical, psychological, and critical perspectives
Robert Kugelmann

CONSTRUCTING PAIN

Historical, Psychological, and Critical Perspectives

Robert Kugelmann

Routledge
Taylor & Francis Group
LONDON AND NEW YORK

First published 2017
by Routledge
2 Park Square, Milton Park, Abingdon, Oxon OX14 4RN

and by Routledge
711 Third Avenue, New York, NY 10017

Routledge is an imprint of the Taylor & Francis Group, an informa business

British Library Cataloguing in Publication Data
A catalogue record for this book is available from the British Library

Library of Congress Cataloging in Publication Data
Names: Kugelmann, Robert, 1948– author.
Title: Constructing pain : historical, psychological and critical perspectives / Robert Kugelmann.
Description: Abingdon, Oxon ; New York, NY : Routledge, 2017.
Identifiers: LCCN 2016029586 | ISBN 9781138841208 (hardback : alk. paper) | ISBN 9781138841222 (pbk. : alk. paper) | ISBN 9781315732367 (e-book)
Subjects: LCSH: Pain—History. | Pain—Physiological aspects. | Pain—Psychological aspects.
Classification: LCC RB127 .K835 2017 | DDC 616/.0472—dc23
LC record available at https://lccn.loc.gov/2016029586

ISBN: 978-1-138-84120-8 (hbk)
ISBN: 978-1-138-84122-2 (pbk)
ISBN: 978-1-315-73236-7 (ebk)

Typeset in Bembo
by Apex CoVantage, LLC

CONTENTS

ACKNOWLEDGMENTS

I thank first of all Antonia Lyons and Kerry Chamberlain, the editors of this series, *Critical Approaches to Health*, for the invitation to write this book. I am grateful to the many members of the International Society of Critical Health Psychology for opportunities to present some of this research and for their critical reception of it. In particular, I thank Michael Murray for his invitation to participate in the first critical health psychology conference in 1999. Without that meeting, this book would never have materialized. I thank my Cheiron colleagues, too numerous to mention, for their suggestions and criticisms over the years. I thank the following students in my Health Psychology class at the University of Dallas in the fall of 2015 for reading the manuscript and providing editorial advice, suggestions, corrections, and improvements: Christen Bounsall, Miranda Eastham, Laura Farrell, Gretchen Geisheker, John Howard, Thomas Kaiser, Natalie Kitten, Celia Miroglio, Leah Nappe, Elizabeth O'Connell, Stephanie Ogbo, Elizabeth Paschall, Rachel Rossi, Andrea Sanchez, and Micah Wood.

The writing of this book has been supported in part by release time from the University of Dallas, including a sabbatical. King-Haggar Faculty Development funds provided me with opportunities to write on and present many of the topics of the book.

I thank the following publishers for permission to use material from previously published articles:

For portions of "Introspective Psychology, Pure and Applied: Henry Rutgers Marshall on Pain and Pleasure." *History of Psychology, 4*, 34–58. Copyright © 2001 by the American Psychological Association. Adapted with permission. The use of this information does not imply endorsement by the publisher.

For portions of "Complaining About Chronic Pain," reprinted from *Social Science and Medicine, 49*(12), 1663–1676, with permission from Elsevier.

SERIES EDITOR PREFACE

Critical approaches to health

Introduction

Health is a major issue for people all around the world and is fundamental to individual well-being, personal achievements, and satisfaction, as well as to families, communities, and societies. It is also embedded in social notions of participation and citizenship. Much has been written about health, from a variety of perspectives and disciplines, but a lot of this writing takes a biomedical and causally positivist approach to health matters, neglecting the historical, social, and cultural contexts and environments within which health is experienced, understood, and practiced. It is an appropriate time to introduce a new series of books that offer critical, social science perspectives on important health topics.

The *Critical Approaches to Health* series aims to provide new critical writing on health by presenting critical, interdisciplinary, and theoretical writing about health, where matters of health are framed quite broadly. The series will include books that range across important health matters, including general health-related issues (such as gender and media), major social issues for health (such as medicalisation, obesity, and palliative care), particular health concerns (such as pain, doctor–patient interaction, health services, and health technologies), particular health problems (such as diabetes, autoimmune disease, and medically unexplained illness), or health for specific groups of people (such as the health of migrants, the homeless, and the aged), or combinations of these.

The series seeks above all to promote critical thought about health matters. By critical, we mean going beyond the critique of the topic and work in the field to more general considerations of power and benefit and, in particular, to addressing concerns about whose understandings and interests are upheld and whose are marginalised by the approaches, findings, and practices in these various domains of health. Such critical agendas involve reflections on what constitutes knowledge, how it is created, and how it is used. Accordingly, critical approaches consider epistemological and theoretical positioning, as well as issues of methodology and practice, and seek to examine how health is enmeshed within broader social relations and structures. Books within this series take up this challenge and seek to provide new insights and understandings by applying a critical agenda to their topics.

In the current book, *Constructing Pain: Historical, Psychological, and Critical Perspectives*, Robert Kugelmann addresses a fundamental issue that pervades health: pain. This book provides a unique perspective on how pain is, can, and should be understood in contemporary life. The opening sections of the book provide the historical context around pain and how a medicalised view of pain came to be increasingly dominant. The book turns from that to exploring personal experiences of pain and to examining pain from a variety of perspectives, including semiotic, phenomenological, discursive, and moral. These chapters show how pain is complex, open to different interpretations and meanings, invoked in identities and subjectivities, and is as much a socially shared as an individual phenomenon. In closing, the book takes us back into the moral order of pain, connecting pain to larger societal concerns of justice, war, and evil. This book considers pain in all its forms and provides a level of scholarly discussion about pain that will leave readers with a host of new understandings on what pain can be.

Kerry Chamberlain and Antonia Lyons
October 2016

INTRODUCTION

To begin, a metaphor: Just as people make love, they also make pain. Lovemaking involves, especially in its older, more circumspect usage, practices and institutions that circumscribe it. The making of love is a natural and cultivated kind of thing. Similarly with pain: Even if the fall into pain is more literal in one sense than the fall into love, the fall still occurs in a social order that has ready-made ways of constructing it. Pain, in its expression, alleviation, and suffering, is a performance that is as personal as cultural, as mental as physical, just as the making of love. We also "do" pain, as Joanna Bourke (2014) has aptly put it. To avoid the ambiguities of make/do, we shall use the more neutral term "construct" – hence the name of this book. Imagine pain to be a kind of building: Natural material, such as wood, is transformed by human knowledge and activity, and a place for inhabitation results. The difference is that few desire to inhabit the house of pain.

Once upon a time, there was no pain. Pain entered the world in a fateful moment. According to Genesis, that moment occurred when Eve and Adam ate the fruit of the tree and gained self-knowledge. According to Hesiod, when Pandora, the beautiful and deceptive gift of the gods to Epimetheus, the hapless brother of Prometheus, opened the box that was best left closed, pain escaped. Evil entered the world. In these accounts, the birth of pain cut humanity off from the Good. In these accounts, how we reckon with pain shapes our lives.

Pain, like eros and death, is a central mystery of life. Pain happens because we are made of flesh and bone: It is part of nature. Pain happens because we have awareness; no sentience, no pain. Pain has a history, a history not only of human responses to this natural thing but also a history of how it is felt, expressed, and addressed. Pain, synonymous with the sense of reality (*pinch me*), is also constructed, changeable – an artifact. Bridging the couplet of nature and culture does not make pain different from other fateful events. A child, a language, a friendship, a delusion: All are both natural and artificial. The human genius is to be a demiurge; we construct things. Cultures and individuals take the materials that lay around and within them and construct things, transforming them in the process. I mean no romantic celebration: Pain can be forged with slavery, torture, war, disease, and industrial economy just as readily as with spiritual yearning for the Other or the hardening of the athlete or the warrior for the contest.

This book explores the constructing of pain in the contemporary world. It is intended as a contribution to critical approaches to health in the human sciences. *Critical* means many things, and in this book it means two things: First, it means questioning the presuppositions of our present understanding of pain as rooted in the medical gaze and the anatomical image of the body. These preconceptions are herein challenged, and the result is an expanded conception of pain. Second, *critical* means a concern for the ethical dimensions of the human sciences, including psychology, sociology, anthropology, and public health. Pain is, above all else, a moral phenomenon. It claims us personally.

There is no single entity of pain. *Pain* exists as *pains*, in the plural. This in itself is not news. The book argues for including pains other than those called physical pains, especially emotional (or mental or psychological) pain and moral pain as genuine pain. An emotional pain is one felt when personal loss occurs, for example. Evil action inflicts moral pain. The topic of moral pain initially surfaced with concerns about war veterans who have been betrayed by their leaders and/or have witnessed, perpetrated, or suffered outrages to their sense of the good. This expanded conception of pain harkens back to a preneurological narrowing of the meaning of pain, as we shall see. The narrative of the book shows, first of all, how pain became constructed narrowly as "real pain" – that is, sensory pain. Then, second of all, the narrative develops an expanded meaning of pain. The book thus seeks to recover older constructions of pain in the context of contemporary understandings.

The book has two sections. The first part examines significant ways in which pain has been constructed from the nineteenth century up to the late twentieth century. It is not meant to be comprehensive; its center is the theme of human embodiment. Chapters 1 and 2 show how the anatomical image of the body became dominant in the conception of pain, first through the introduction of anesthetics and painkillers and then through the ways in which the study of the nervous system in relation to pain narrowed the meaning of pain to sensory pain. We live in the world that ether institutionalized but did not create. Incredibly quickly, metaphorical connotations of ether and chloroform were exploited, especially for humor, indicating that these substances signified more than a useful and beneficial tool for surgeons. Anesthesia symbolized, among other things, modern comforts and willful ignorance of suffering.

Pain underwent a number of transformations, including its articulation in discourses that established the utility and meaninglessness of pain, and the promise of its elimination with the development of anesthetics and other drugs for its alleviation. For us, pain is something that can be prevented or eliminated. This is the great divide separating us from the past. It is not simply that we have power over pain that earlier generations did not know. Anesthetics and painkillers transformed existential possibilities. Have these changes made us less tolerant of any pain whatsoever, or have they been an answer to an enduring yearning? We explore the charge that we moderns suffer from algophobia, irrational fear of pain. What that charge indicates is a growing meaningless of pain on the one hand – the so-called secularization of pain – and, on the other hand, a sense that these new substances mean that we have achieved real progress. What emerged is a sense that pain ought not to last, that acute pain is the prototype of pain.

Anesthesia helped burn into the modern psyche the medical gaze and the anatomical image of the body, which proved to be so compelling and fateful for the construction of pain in the late nineteenth century. It made for the appearance of "real pain," which threw all other pains into the sphere of the imaginary, into the mind. In the late nineteenth century, psychologists debated the nature of pain. Some of the antagonists represented the sensation theory, which held that pain is a sensation mediated by the firing of peripheral nerve endings signaling tissue damage. Their opponents paired pleasure with pain and viewed them both as qualities of mental states of all kinds, not only sensory events. The sensation theory carried the day. The outcome of this struggle was the narrowing of pain to "real pain," pain caused by the stimulation of peripheral nerves. The sensation theory dominated medicine and psychology until the 1960s, when pain was reconsidered in light of criticisms of the inherent dualism in the concept of real pain.

Chapter 3 turns to the beginning of the undoing of sensory pain as the only "real pain," with critiques from within psychology and related fields of "dualism" in the constructing of pain. In the mid-twentieth century, objections over the implications of real pain – notably the tendency to dismiss psychogenic pains – became paramount. By the middle of the twentieth century, doubts accumulated about the sensation theory of pain. Three different criticisms of so-called Cartesian dualism appeared: the gate control theory, the redefinition of pain as an unpleasant experience, and the category of pain behavior. The significance of these criticisms was that they marked a return of subjectivity to the psychological conception of pain.

After exploring the history of modern constructions of pain, we turn to a phenomenology of pain in order to overcome the limitations of the anatomical image of the body through the phenomenological notion of embodied subjectivity. We investigate one of the distinctly modern ways of being in pain – chronic pain – through its social representations and the terms in which it is experienced. Social representations of chronic pain, drawn primarily from newspaper accounts, show the ways in which the neurological and psychological concepts of pain enter common-sense discourse and action. The exploration of social representations also indicates the major conflict over chronic pain: the place of drugs. Following this first part come interpretations of narratives of individuals in a pain management program. Discursive formations emerged in those interviews that complement social representations of chronic pain. Finally, and drawing on a distinction made by Emmanuel Levinas, the chapter concludes by turning from what is said to the saying of it – that is, to speech addressed by Others, to pleas that insist upon justice. Chronic pain proves to be a type of moral pain.

Chronic pain is a type of pain that acts contrary to what we expect. We ordinarily expect pain to end after a period of time. I believe that we have this expectation not only because, empirically, that is what usually happens but also because we "remember" the Golden Age and long for it with nostalgia. Chronic pain, however, is often endless in the experience of those who suffer from it, and it often defies standard medical treatments.

Then we turn to everyday pain, which includes psychological as well as physical pains. Narratives of pain, regardless of their alleged cause (a broken bone or a broken heart), have similar forms and plots. In both types of narratives, the pain is felt, even if not in the anatomical image of the body. These narratives involve a "fall" out of a shared world. There emerges a desire for something else that proves to be the key moment. To be sure, we construct everyday pain in the shadow of biomedicine, which accentuates the differences.

A phenomenological conception of pain is, at this point, ripe for the picking, and we develop the concept of pain as an attunement, as a felt bodily sense. Phenomenologically understood, pain is a kind of active passivity. Pain of any sort confounds our dichotomies, asserting and contradicting them simultaneously: Pain is an *it*, pain is *I*; pain isolates me from the social world, pain exposes me, leaves me vulnerable, throbbing with every insult and look of scorn. A study of phenomenologies of pain follows an integration of "physical" and "mental" pain, with the conclusion that pain is, in Heideggerian terms, an attunement, a mode of being in the world that places us on the edge of existence. As such, pain is not a pure passivity; it is also an activity, even if it is enacted despite what we want. Pain reveals the disturbances, the ruptures, the brokenness of the world and of ourselves.

Pain as attunement can be recast and furthered by considering pain as a sign, following Charles Sanders Peirce's semiotics. What pain as a sign allows us to see is that pain is a way of knowing ourselves and our existence. Semiotics shows how we construct pain and construct ourselves with pain.

In the final chapter, we conclude not with solutions to the problem of pain but with pain as a way of apprehending the real. Expanding our conception of pain to the moral realm, pain as a way of knowing can be found especially in the suffering of evil. In pain, we know evil. To develop this notion further, we turn to contexts in which pain opens up the world. In the "moral injuries" of war and other forms of injustice, we see how being in pain exposes people to the tragic, the horrible, the evils of existence.

Reference

Bourke, J. (2014). *The story of pain: From prayer to painkillers.* Oxford, England: Oxford University Press.

PART I
Constructing pain historically

This part of the book examines several distinct moments in the construction of pain in the modern world. To begin, there is the development of anesthetics in the nineteenth century. The context in which they were used is as important as the substances themselves. The context was medical. When physicians used anesthetics, they were applying them to the body understood anatomically, as an object for treatment. As a result of the widespread acceptance of anesthetics, the anatomical image of the body became socially relevant as never before. This is important because, phenomenologically speaking, anatomy gives *a* truth about the body, not *the* truth. Ether and its kin promised "the death of pain," as the neurologist and poet, Silas Weir Mitchell, hoped on the fiftieth anniversary of its first use. In the wake of this transformation of the experience of pain, with analgesics and anesthetics promising an end to pain, was the understanding that pain was ideally acute: here today and gone tomorrow.

Following this transformation, the late nineteenth century constructed "real pain" – that is, sensory pain associated with the stimulation of nerve endings in the anatomical body's periphery. Other pain not conforming to this prototype became somehow less than real. In the middle of the twentieth century, this sensation theory of pain came under fire as Cartesian. We find three ways in which the notion of pain was broadened: the gate control theory, the operationalized definition of pain, and the notion of pain behavior. These more contemporary ways of constructing pain open up to phenomenological considerations, which Part II shall address.

1

CONSTRUCTING MODERN PAIN

"The conquest of pain"

Anesthetics and painkillers transformed the existential possibilities for the experience of pain and what people do about it. These innovations of the nineteenth century built upon earlier developments. The most significant of these is discussed in the following section.

The anatomical image of the body

Even though anatomy had been practiced for several centuries, a humoral image of the body still held sway in the eighteenth century. That began to change by the turn of the nineteenth century, and "the study of anatomy, both theoretical and practical, was seen as the cornerstone of all medical teaching" (Bonner, 1995, p. 142). Anatomical images of the body also served to differentiate an emerging medical profession from that of other practitioners, as Stelmackowich (2012) indicates in a discussion of the development of illustrated medical textbooks at the beginning of the nineteenth century: "These new diagrams and illustrations constituted new visual and discursive practices and were crucial in developing the professional and institutionalized discipline of medicine" (p. 51). In addition to the study of anatomy, and perhaps even more important, was a new concentration on "morbid anatomy" or pathology. Initiation into pathology, whereby the innards became visual objects – in contrast to the fluxes and flows of the humoral body – became "the prerequisite for a medical career" (Stelmackowich, 2012, p. 52).

With the introduction early in the century of the stethoscope, the patient's silence, rather than his or her narrative (Reiser, 1978), became an increasingly established part of the "medical gaze," to use Michel Foucault's (1973) term for the visualization of disease in the anatomical image. This image – the corpse opened up anatomically – became the royal road to knowledge of the living body. Whereas today such knowledge is assumed, it is important to signal what an innovation this type of knowing was. Phenomenological studies of the history of this change (Bishop, 2011; Duden, 1991; van den Berg, 1972) show that the anatomical image meant an alienation from the flesh of the living being; Romanyshyn (1989) calls the anatomical image the "abandoned body" – that is, the body of no one. Before the medical gaze and its abandoned body, physicians relied on patient narratives in order to interpret what was wrong with the patient's health. In Illich's (2005) words, earlier medical discourse focused on the question "how is that 'who' who you are today" (pp. 125–126). That is, the question asked about the person's story of who he or she was. It asked about embodied living. Illich calls this embodied living the "felt body," the body that the person is. The anatomical image promises better know-how in treating illness, but this technological advantage has come at a price. In some measure, this book is a study of the consequences of the anatomical image for the construction of pain.

For many people living at the time when the abandoned body was becoming the ground of medicine, this alienation was felt deeply. Into the nineteenth century, dissection was punishment added to execution – and often more feared because of the ways in which the Christian teaching on the resurrection of the dead was understood: "People viewed dissection as a desecration of the corpse and believed that it would impede resurrection and deny the survival of identity after death. While execution was a threat to one's life, dissection was an assault on one's soul" (Hulkower, 2011, p. 23). Only in the 1830s did American states begin to pass legislation authorizing the use of unclaimed dead paupers for dissection. Legislation for the donation of one's body after death – changing what had been punishment into a gift of the living – occurred only after 1968 (p. 25). Earlier, with the demand for cadavers exceeding the supply, the crime of "body snatching" was profitable, leading to such incidents as a riot in New York City in 1788, with mobs sacking hospitals and kidnapping medical students (p. 24). In 1828, the trial of William Burke and William Hare took place; Burke and Hare found that murder provided a more ready supply of fresh corpses than grave robbing. They were convicted and executed for murder. This infamous pair had an indirect connection with the physician who will serve as our occasional witness to the changes that occurred in the nineteenth century: Benjamin Ward Richardson (1828–1896).

A representative of the time of transition

Throughout this chapter, we will have occasion to draw on Richardson's testimony. He was a British physician who contributed significantly to medicine and public health. He does not represent everyone involved in the story of the transformation of pain, but he did witness some of the key changes. He was a medical student in 1846, the year that surgical anesthesia was first used to wide acclaim in Boston, and he witnessed the transition to painless surgery firsthand. He started medical studies at Anderson University in Glasgow in 1845; in addition to pursuing anatomical studies there, he also attended a course on the anatomy of the brain given by Robert Knox. Richardson praised Knox's knowledge of anatomy, although Knox had been vilified because he had bought cadavers from Burke and Hare. Knox had not been prosecuted, but life in Edinburgh had become uncomfortable, and he left town. Suffice it to say, Richardson acquired the medical gaze in his studies with Knox. He did not finish medical school in Glasgow (a result of his own illness), and he completed medical studies at St. Andrews. He later moved to London, becoming a member of the Royal Academy of Physicians in 1857 and a fellow in 1865 (Wallis, 2004).

The abolition of pain: anesthetics as substance and symbol

The psychological philosopher Alexander Bain brought together the British empiricist tradition, which conceptualized the human mind in terms of sensations and their associations, and the emerging physiological psychology. In discussing the "emotions of action," Bain (1859) used the term *anæsthesia* to refer to ways of allaying "mental excitement" (p. 186, note). The term was new: "I have gladly adopted the term 'anæsthesia' into the phraseology of mental science" (p. 188, note). In the pursuit of some goal, we can experience anæsthesia, or "the quieting of consciousness," because of our rapt attention. Bain mentioned other anesthetic means, mental and physical, including the "important additions derived from the recent introduction of Ether and Chloroform" (p. 187, note). Bain affirmed the view that all societies have their chemical means of altering consciousness: "Alcohol, Tobacco, Tea, Opium, Hemp, Betel, and the other narcotics, are the resort of millions, for the production of mental elation, or soothing irritation and pain" (p. 235). For Bain, anesthetic action was a natural process that had recently seen chemical enhancement with the introduction of ether, chloroform, and nitrous oxide.

Nitrous oxide and ether had been used prior to 1846, and not only by the romantic poets Coleridge and Southey, who inhaled nitrous oxide in the 1790s (Papper, 1995). There had been public exhibits of nitrous oxide, with the public invited to inhale, and the British artist "Robert Seymour . . . in 1830 . . . portrayed the forcible use of laughing gas as a remedy for nagging wives" (Pernick, 1985, p. 86). Nitrous oxide, synthesized by Joseph Priestly in 1772, had been used as an intoxicant since 1799. Ether, on the other hand, had been around for centuries. It too was used as an intoxicant, either inhaled or drunk; its first surgical use was by a dentist, William Thomas Green Morton, in 1846. Nitrous oxide came into surgical use a bit later, ether and chloroform being preferred.

The term *anesthesia* was fairly new, although it was used before Bain incorporated it into psychological discourse. Halttunen (1995) writes that "in the early eighteenth century, the term 'anesthesia' had referred to a defective lack of feeling; by the end of the century, it had come to connote a 'positive medical relieving of feeling, a blessing rather than a defect'" (p. 310). That meaning was further refined. According to Stanley (2003), "the term 'anaesthesia' seems to have been first used in 1833 when the *Lancet* published a translation of a French article discussing the condition of 'diminution, or total loss, of bodily sensation' with a view, ironically, to its cure" (p. 285). Thus, before the actual introduction of surgical anesthesia, the idea and the term were in circulation.

The introduction of surgical anesthesia

The introduction of surgical anesthesia in 1846 was one of those events that stand out as forever changing the human condition. Morris (1991) writes that anesthetics "transformed our cultural assumptions about pain" (p. 64). Anesthetics symbolize the rift between our experience of pain and that of those who lived before the mid-nineteenth century. The ground had, however, been long prepared, and anesthetics materialized a change in cultural evaluations of pain that had appeared earlier, with the rise of a culture of "sensibility" in the English-speaking world: "The eighteenth-century cult of sensibility redefined pain as unacceptable and indeed eradicable and thus opened the door to a new revulsion from pain, which, though later regarded as 'instinctive' and 'natural,' has in fact proved to be distinctly modern" (Halttunen, 1995, p. 304). Halttunen claims that "middle-class sensitivity to pain" "contributed to the late eighteenth-century intensification of medical efforts to discover an effective form of anesthesia" (p. 309). In this stress on the sympathetic viewing of the pain and suffering of others, pain became obscene, simultaneously intolerable and exciting.

The events of the 1840s, then, presuppose an ongoing shift in cultural values, making more urgent the elimination of what was no longer tolerable. Crawford Williamson Long, a Georgia dentist, first used ether surgically in 1842 (Dormandy, 2006). But Long was not well connected, and Morton's demonstration of the surgical use of ether in a Boston medical classroom in 1846 proved to be decisive in getting anesthesia circulating in the medical community at home and abroad. The fame of anesthetics for surgery spread rapidly, not only because their effectiveness had been demonstrated but also because the means for rapid diffusion were available by ship, by railroad, by telegraph, and by newspaper. Before the end of 1847, surgeons in Britain, France, Germany, and Australia employed surgical anesthesia. In his memoirs, Benjamin Ward Richardson (1897) recalled that while he was a medical student in Glasgow,

> news came from America by the ship *Arcadia* that the abolition of pain had been made manifest there in the operating theatre at Boston, U.S.A. In London, Liston, following up the plan of Wells, Morton, and Jackson, had removed a limb painlessly by letting the patient previously breathe the vapour of ether, and we were soon to see the advantages of this immortal advance in the profession of medicine, the most striking advance, probably, that the world has ever witnessed.
>
> *(p. 78)*

This "immortal advance" altered the existential possibilities for pain in our lives.

News of the new way of performing surgery spread quickly. By early 1847, American newspapers were reporting on Morton's demonstration of ether. The Vermont abolitionist newspaper *The Voice of Freedom* published "Inhalation of Ethereal Vapor" (1847, January 7), picking up John C. Warren's account from the *Boston Medical and Surgical Journal* of December 6, 1846. Early 1847 saw similar newspaper accounts across the country. After Simpson used chloroform in November 1847 in Edinburgh, that report also spread across the United States. In "Chloroform" (1848, January 28), the *Vermont Phoenix* reported Simpson's discovery and quoted from the *Boston Olive Branch*, which "requested Dr Hitchcock, Dentist of this city, to furnish us with a report of some of the cases connected with the success of its application" (p. 3). Hitchcock included testimony from the Rev. Mr. S., who had several teeth and roots removed:

> I called on Dr Hitchcock, who administered the vapor of fifteen or twenty drops of the Chloroform, and extracted the teeth without producing the least pain. – The time employed in the whole operation did not exceed thirty seconds. While inhaling it, I experienced scarcely any uneasiness. No unpleasant effects followed its influence.
>
> *(p. 3)*

The Vermont article concluded by pointing out that "Dr. Putnam, of this village, we understand, administers the Chloroform successfully" (p. 3). By February 1848, the *New York Daily Tribune* ("Chloroform," 1848, February 8) carried an advertisement for the sale of chloroform to physicians and druggists.

As with most new technologies, conflicting views surfaced. In a letter to the *Journal of Commerce*, a New York dentist, Horace Kimball, one of the first to use anesthetics (Morrison & Sharples, 1897, p. 664), wrote in support of "lethêon gas," Morton's name for ether. Kimball (1846) took issue with Richard S. Kissam, Jr., a well-regarded New York surgeon, who objected

> to the "inhalation of narcotic vapors" – because, as he says, the sensation of pain (which such inhalation completely destroys,) has been given us to stimulate and set in action the recuperative process of the organization, after injuries," and therefore it is desirable that patients should be left to feel pain which is naturally endured under surgical operations.
>
> *(p. 22)*

Kimball's letter was reprinted in a circular that Morton published himself to promote his claim to priority (Osler, 1929, p. 135).

This new form of sleep raised other anxieties, which also haunted hypnosis – namely, that untoward things could happen to someone under the influence. A brief piece in *Punch* ("The New Discovery in Surgery," 1847) portrayed a common anxiety of the time: "A man may, it seems, have his legs cut from under him without his knowing it." Pernick (1985) found that one objection to anesthesia was that it threatened "the loss of the patient's supervisory power over the operation" (p. 58), a concern echoed in the *Punch* article. Richardson's (1897) fellow students expressed the same anxiety. One volunteered

> like a valiant young martyr, for experiment, and allowing his enthusiastic *confrères* to put him into the deepest ethereal sleep for the sake of practice; and I remember that when he came to himself again he looked about him, as if he expected that, for the sake of practice, some one might have lightened him of a limb or two while he sat an unconscious and helpless victim.
>
> *(p. 86)*

Kissam's attitude is one that sounds foreign to those of us who take comfort in the assurance of anesthetic operations, so it is worthwhile to look at his objections. There were medical reasons to avoid anesthesia, and not only because of complications and death resulting from it. A leading American physician wrote of pain: "The actions of life are maintained by it. Were it not for the stimulation induced by pain, most surgical operations would be followed by dissolution" (John P. Harrison, quoted in Pernick, 1985, p. 125). A patient in pain, screaming even, was a patient alive: "Pain was the most powerful and valuable stimulant. Many a brave soldier seemingly dead was brought back from the brink by the feel of the surgeon's steel" (Dormandy, 2006, p. 283). Pain helped speed healing after surgery, according to some physicians. In addition, there were cultural norms celebrating the endurance of pain and religious objections to the avoidance of pain: "In Milan Cardinal Berlusconi . . . delivered a much-quoted sermon in which he castigated those who sought to abolish the pain of surgery, 'one of the Almighty's most merciful provisions'" (Dormandy, 2006, p. 198). However, believers lined up on both sides of the debate.

Surgery before and after ether

A sense of the difference that surgical anesthetics made in the experience of pain can be garnered from descriptions of surgery from the time just before and just after their introduction. Since the patient is "asleep" with the administration of ether and its kin, we will look at accounts from the point of view of the surgeon. Our informant, Benjamin Ward Richardson, was a public health reformer and a researcher in anesthesia:

> He was highly productive, discovering fourteen new anaesthetics, several of which were soon widely used . . . and inventing the first double-valved mouthpiece for the administration of chloroform. He also invented the ether spray, the only known method of local anaesthesia until the introduction of the topical use of cocaine in 1884. In addition he investigated the potential of mesmerism, electricity, and other possible alternatives to chemical anaesthetics.
>
> *(Wallis, 2004)*

Late in life, Richardson (1897) penned his life story, *Vita Medica.* He described his initiation into surgery:

> I recall that when I had to witness the first capital operation I sought the companionship of a student much older than myself, but it turned out that he was more nervous than I. . . . I made up my mind to face the ordeal bravely, and for a time was quite taken out of myself by seeing the consummate calmness and dexterity with which the operator – the late Professor Lawrie – proceeded in his painful task. . . . [S]uch was the rapidity in this case the operation was actually over, in so far as the major part of it was concerned, before the patient uttered a single cry. If all had stopped there, all had been well; but just at that moment, as if giving vent to a long-suppressed agony, the patient uttered a scream, and, in spite of the tenderness and firmness with which the nurses assured him it was all over, continued to scream and struggle, so that he had to be securely held whilst the final steps of the operation were performed. Some of my comrades, neophytes like myself, became faint, and some left the theatre. I kept my legs, saw in a kind of haze the man being carried away, but soon came back to thorough consciousness. Several weeks went over my head before composure of mind accompanied such scenes as these. I think we all got hardened at last, but it was not permanent hardening. If we were away a few times from the scene, we had a return of the terror, in a minor degree, so soon as we resumed work.
>
> *(pp. 79–80)*

This passage was written after Richardson's research on anesthetics, and its rhetorical work was to display the horrors of pre-anesthetic surgery, in a passage that displayed great sensibility. Nevertheless, the account described an initiation ritual, since the point of this witnessing was to prepare him to perform surgery. What filled him with terror were the screams and the struggles of the patient, who was inconsolable in his agony. The patient's pain filled the room, leaving Richardson anxious in the presence of this violence perpetrated in the name of healing. In what to modern eyes looks like bitter irony, Richardson recalled:

> When I asked my first practical teacher how he thought I should get through the ordeal of seeing and taking part in an operation, he replied that, as in learning to smoke, time brought tolerance, but that a man must keep his hand in if he meant to retain his firmness and presence of mind.
>
> *(pp. 78–79)*

The contrast between Richardson's sensibility and the unsentimental attitude toward pain of his elder, who viewed surgical pain as inevitable, could not be clearer.

How reliable a witness was Richardson? Pernick (1985) found that at least some physicians shared the attitude Richardson described, in that "operating on screaming, pain-ravaged people took its toll on surgeons as well as on their clients"

(p. 82). Others, described by the Confederate physician Julian John Chisholm (1861) as "older surgeons," heard "the cries of the patient as music to the ear" (p. 381). Chisholm himself recommended the use of chloroform for all serious surgery. Yet for those older surgeons, pain signaled that the patient was alive. They saw pain as stimulating the body's own curative processes. Moreover, pain promoted endurance and good character. Pernick (pp. 198–201) found some evidence of a generational difference in the use of anesthetics by surgeons, thus supporting the implication of what Richardson described.

Patients, too, had mixed feelings about surgical pain. While anesthesia meant that many who had previously avoided an operation out of dread of pain would now consent, others feared the loss of "supervisory power" (Pernick, 1985, p. 58) that anesthetics entailed. Then there were fears of death from anesthesia itself, a not-unwarranted concern. Patients insisted on anesthesia, however, and the increasing use of anesthetics was driven in part by demand as well as by surgeons' attitudes.

Before anesthesia, the surgeon had often interacted with the patient upon whom he was operating. Richardson (1897) praised the courage of many of his patients – the endurance of pain meant strength of character – but, at times, other measures were necessary:

> We often endeavoured to divert the attention of sufferers towards another subject, as a mother is seen to divert the attention of a child, in pain or in fear, towards some glittering thing or something entirely new, and here we experienced what the mother experiences – that is to say, we either made matters better or worse.
>
> *(pp. 80–81)*

Maternal solicitude, and the passive helplessness of the patient, marked the surgical relationship. Richardson described how, on the operating table, the patient would at first submit to the procedure with "a kind of holy courage" until the

> suffering began, upon which there was an almost certain change of view, and insistence, of the strongest kind at first, that the operation should be stopped at all risks; a resistance which had to be gently but resolutely overcome, followed, when resistance was useless, by as energetic a request for the proceedings to finish as rapidly as possible.
>
> *(p. 81)*

Here, one sees the surgeon, knowingly inflicting torment on a person who asks for the suffering to cease, persuading the patient to submit.

Richardson (1897) contrasted these recollections with the first demonstration of surgery with ether in dramatic form. Richardson's professor told the students "of a method by which the most important operations could be performed while the patient undergoing the operation was asleep" (pp. 83–84). The class rushed to the operating theater of the Royal Infirmary. The theater was used as a chapel on Sunday, and Richardson "got into the pulpit, which formed an excellent place for observation," a location otherwise off limits for the medical students "except on such a memorable day" (p. 84). Andrew Buchanan was to perform the operation, prefacing the procedure with "the news that had come from the Massachusetts Hospital, explaining that the process consisted in laying the patient in deep sleep by the inhalation of the vapour of ether" (p. 84). Richardson then described the other main character:

> The patient was then sent for, and came in with quite a smiling face, delighted with the idea of being cut without pain, and rather proud, I fancy, at being the first man in Scotland selected to enjoy the honour as well as the pleasure.
>
> *(pp. 84–85)*

The patient – Richardson thought his name was Macleod – agreed to the procedure and was instructed to breathe ether vapor from a sponge. Macleod at first acted intoxicated, recited some Robbie Burns,

> then lapsed into perfect quietude, and soon afterward was allowed to wake up with the operation completed, not knowing that he had passed through anything more than a curious dream, feeling, as he affirmed with a broad grin, just "a wee bit fou," and in no degree ashamed of his acquaintanceship with that condition.
>
> *(p. 85)*

The paternalistic phrasing notwithstanding, this account marked a strong contrast with the previous one. Where there had been an intense relationship between surgeon and patient, marked by dread on both sides, here there was the sense of relief on both sides.

Richardson described the introduction of anesthesia as "the abolition of pain" (p. 87), using a word also associated with the end of slavery. In fact, Richardson described his public health work as an effort "for the abolition of disease," a work as "earnest" as the fight for the "abolition of slavery" (p. 247). This association between pain and slavery illustrates the ethical grounding of the introduction of anesthetics and how they symbolized moral progress. Richardson's descriptions served to show that the introduction of surgical anesthesia was the equivalent of the elimination of an evil, analogous to the end of slavery – with progress would come freedom from the oppression of pain.

Anesthesia as metaphor and social representation

The first etherized patients were barely awake when anesthesia began to be used metaphorically. Significant examples occurred in *Punch, or the London Charivari.*

This satirical magazine, founded in 1841, had broad appeal among middle-class readers in Britain and the United States. Queen Victoria and Members of Parliament read it (Altick, 1997, p. 17); the *Times* (London) reprinted some of its stories; and this periodical, which "sought its market in the generally conservative middle class" (Altick, 1997, p. xix), had wide circulation by 1847. It helped shape social representations of anesthesia, in part by humorously exaggerating its significations. First, the literal action of the drugs was praised:

> A bladder of Ether, oh! Fill for me!
> Let those who prefer it feel pain;
> but I'll have out my tooth, though a molar it be,
> And it never shall plague me again.
> The dentist his forceps displays to my eye,
> I feel no emotions distressing;
> Inhaling my Ether, the wrench I defy –
> Oh! ether indeed is a blessing!
>
> *("The Blessing of Ether," 1847)*

Another poem, "The Blessings of Chloroform" (1848) used hyperbole to depict the virtues of this new substance, for now we could be "flay'd alive, unconscious of a feeling of uneasiness." Unlike early newspaper accounts that propagated this new knowledge, the articles in *Punch* made anesthetics familiar by comparing them to alcohol and by reminding readers of their earlier uses for their intoxicating effects. That is, much of the humor turned on similarities between anesthesia and alcohol on the one hand and on multiple meanings of "insensibility" on the other. Anesthesia, in practice and in discourse, quickly entered the vernacular.

Almost immediately, observers saw anesthetics as symbols for the general elimination of pain from life. Suggested uses of ether extended its pain-alleviating abilities to other social situations of suffering, such as transforming a nagging wife's scolding into "a most beautiful dream" ("Wonderful Effects," 1847, p. 60). The uses of chloroform were extended to anything that causes a person any pain whatsoever, including emotional pain:

> When some vile dun with his little bill is vexing you;
> When the Tax Collector's knock assails your door;
> When aught is troubling, annoying, or perplexing you;
> When, in short, you're plagued with any kind of bore,
> Do not rage and fume and fret, behaving with stupidity,
> Take the matter quietly with coolness and placidity;
> Don't indulge in conduct and in language reprehensible –
> Snuff a little Chloroform, be prudent, and insensible.
>
> *("The Blessings of Chloroform," 1848)*

Painlessness rendered one insensitive in other ways. *Punch* declared that a railway company had

> resolved, that as it is advisable to stop the complaints of the public as much as possible on account of the numerous accidents which, somehow, will occur on the best-regulated railways, rooms be immediately prepared in every station, where persons who dislike being hurt or injured, or are foolishly apprehensive of danger, may have the option of inhaling the ether, so that they may have the privilege of remaining during the whole journey in a state of insensibility, for which act of accommodation the Directors trust the public will be duly thankful.
>
> *("Painless Operation," 1847)*

The irony was that such passengers were to be made insensitive to the real dangers of railway travel. The promise of anesthesia also entailed anxiety about its use.

Positive assessment of surgical anesthesia was but one aspect of a general attitude: Anesthesia made life livable. Along came anesthesia as compensating respite not only to the dangers of railway and industrial accidents but also to the "wear and tear of modern life." *Punch* observed, in other words, what has been termed *algophobia*, or fear of pain, in the social world.

Painkillers

Anesthetics were not the only chemical means to attack pain. Analgesics, or painkillers, were appearing, and they were in high demand in the marketplace. As Pernick (1985) writes:

> The year before the discovery of anesthesia, another almost forgotten breakthrough occurred – the discovery by America's patent medicine industry of the lucrative market for general pain cures. In 1845, Morton's fellow New Englander Perry Davis registered his "Celebrated Pain Killer" trademark and thereby christened an entirely new concept in patent drugs. Unlike most previous nostrums, supposedly good for a variety of *diseases*, Davis' Pain Killer seems to have been the first nationally advertised remedy specifically for *pain*.
>
> *(p. 72; italics in the original)*

Patent medicine companies were the first to advertise nationally, using the expanding medium of the newspaper to sell their wares. This intersection of popular medicine and advertising isolated pain as something capable of being eliminated. As religious assessments of pain declined (Bourke, 2014), pain became increasingly pointless.

A plethora of patent remedies laced with opiates, alcohol, ether, or nitrous oxide – and, later, the chemical synthesis of other compounds – was available in the late nineteenth century in the United States, where "proprietary drugs" were marketed extensively. Only in the early twentieth century was federal legislation enacted to limit supplies. The nineteenth century witnessed a veritable drug revolution. In 1806, Sertürner described morphine, isolated from opium; in 1855, Wood used the newly invented hypodermic needle for injections of morphine to relieve neuralgic pains (Dormandy, 2006, p. 258). The same year, Gaedecke isolated cocaine (Bonica, 1953, p. 167), although it was named 5 years later by Niemann (Schiller, 1990, p. 44). In 1874, Bartholow used chloroform to treat trigeminal neuralgia, the first use of anesthesia for nonsurgical pain (Bonica, 1953, p. 171). In 1884, Koller demonstrated the local anesthetic effect of cocaine – and this was the birth of regional anesthesia (Bonica, 1953, p. 167). That same year, Halsted and Hall, reading Koller's paper, performed the first nerve block prior to surgical and dental interventions (Bonica, 1953, p. 168). Also in this century came amyl nitrate; bromine; chloral hydrate; heroin; and aspirin, a brand name coined by the Bayer Company late in the 1800s.

Fundamental to these changes was the transformation of the production of drugs into an industrial enterprise. Prior to the mid-nineteenth century, the making of drugs was small scale and local for the most part; if drugs were compounded by American pharmacists, for example, this was done in the drugstore's own laboratory (Sonnedecker, 1976, p. 294). The growth of proprietary medicines, such as the numerous painkillers, marked one departure from this traditional way of making drugs; the other was the emergence of the pharmaceutical industry. Two important pain-related products of this alliance between chemistry and industry were heroin (synthesized in 1898) and aspirin (1899).

Drugs changed in other ways, too. A long tradition was ending as the Hippocratic–Galenic understanding of medications gave way to chemical elaborations of the medical gaze:

> New explanatory models were brought to bear on traditional remedies. As the alkaloid was extracted from the complex chemical matrix of plant material, its effects and uses were redefined; not as adjusting system balances of humours and bodily fluids, but as targeting specific organs or tissues, in response to specific individual diseases and performing, ideally, a single beneficial effect.
>
> *(Acker, 1995, p. 116)*

That is, chemical action was coordinated with the anatomical image of the body.

There were also mass movements to restrict the use of such substances. Richardson (1897) recalled how, when he was a young physician, applicants for life insurance who were teetotalers were viewed with suspicion, and he himself would not have recommended them as good risks. Richardson, one among many, turned against the use of alcohol, a result, he said, of his own laboratory investigations. He stated that alcohol should be used sparingly and only with a physician's prescription. In the United States, the temperance movement, aligned variously with the abolitionist and suffrage movements, finally succeeded in establishing Prohibition in 1919 (repealed in 1933). The noun *addict* appeared in 1909, adding a denotation referring to the habit of using morphine and its kin. Fear of addiction, especially when the drugs in question were associated with despised minorities in the eyes of American legislators (opium with the Chinese; cocaine with Southern blacks), helped propel restrictive laws, especially the Harrison Act of 1914 (see Musto, 1999). The result of these changes was that as pain became increasingly meaningless, addiction or the pursuit of painkilling became increasingly feared. There were inherent contradictions in the social representations of pain and its treatment. The possibilities for living were changing socially.

Algophobia?

There is a controversial thesis that states that in the modern world, there has been a decline in the willingness to endure pain, a condition called *algophobia.* The term *algophobia* first appeared in 1897, the year that Bayer began investigating acetylsalicylic acid (aspirin). Some physicians and moralists in the nineteenth century argued that with civilization came greater sensitivity of the nervous system, making us feel pain more acutely. Primitive people are more insensitive: "In the ideology of slave owners [in the United States], it was a commonplace that slaves were relatively insensitive to pain" (Armstrong, 2012, p. 146). Evolutionary thought reinforced this view: "It is now a well-established conclusion of science that the higher we rise in the scale of nervous organization the greater the possibilities of pain" ("The Meaning of Pain," 1906, p. 699). The phenomenological physiologist F.J.J. Buytendijk (1962) declared that moderns, with the advances in medicine that reduce our exposure to pain, suffer from an "immoderate state of algophobia" (p. 16). The phenomenological philosopher Arne Johan Vetlesen (2009) seconds this thesis:

> My assertion is that we, people living in one of the world's most affluent countries, have in the present age developed a conception of pain's position in human life that is possibly the most negative ever. . . . [T]his negative experience is not as obvious and not as spontaneous as we tend to believe. To be more precise, what is not obvious is that the negativity of pain is exclusively to be judged as negative.
>
> *(pp. 8–9)*

As an empirical question, the thesis of algophobia is impossible to evaluate. What did change in the nineteenth century were the possibilities for existence: With anesthesia and painkillers came the expectation that pain could be mastered.

It is not a question of a loss of appetite for inflicting pain, as the products of the defense industry and justifications of torture by political leaders bear witness. It is rather that the position of pain in a hierarchy of values and in relation to power has changed. For Buytendijk, the increased painfulness of pain results from the loss of meaning of pain. But pain had not become meaningless; it was changing its place in a system of values, becoming a scandal.

Increased sensitivity to pain?

René Leriche (1939), the French surgeon who contributed to an understanding of chronic pain, held that moderns are more physiologically sensitive to pain than were people in earlier times. However, he made an epistemological claim, not a moral or biological one. We have trained our senses for acuity so that "we appreciate much more clearly than our predecessors the most subtle differences in things" (p. 54). The means for this training were the improved creature comforts of modernity: "We try to avoid the slightest pain, however fleeting it is, because we know that we have the means of doing so" (p. 54). In other terms, "increased sensitivity" means that there are more possibilities today to avoid pain and to reduce it once it occurs. This availability changes expectations about what ought to happen with pain in the future. This point will lead us to significantly revise the meaning of algophobia.

Pain rendered increasingly avoidable becomes meaningless. If a person does not avail himself or herself of means to alleviate pain, then that is not an expression of patience; it looks foolish or eccentric. No one disputes the meaningfulness of sudden, acute pain. But with chronic pain, the picture changes. Leriche (1939) helped define chronic pain's pointlessness:

> What, then, is physical pain, apart from the circumstances of its production? A dreadful specialized phenomenon, and not a law of Nature. A phenomenon of disease. A disorder whose consequences we must not allow ourselves to regard with indifference, with which we must never compromise, and about which we must try to learn all we can in order the more effectively to counteract it.
>
> *(p. 491)*

Such pain is not "natural" because it serves no useful biological purpose. He had in mind the pains of neuralgias, phantom limb pain, and pain associated with cancer and other chronic diseases. Weir Mitchell (1900) voiced a similar concern in 1896 regarding pain in surgery:

> What purpose hath it? Nay, thy quest is vain:
> Earth hath no answer. If the baffled brain
> Cries, 'T is to warn, to punish – ah, refrain!
> When writhes the child beneath the surgeon's hand,
> What soul shall hope that pain to understand?
> Lo! Science falters o'er the hopeless task,
> And Love and Faith in vain an answer ask,
> When thrilling nerves demand what good is wrought
> Where torture clogs the very source of thought.
>
> *(p. 16)*

Acute pain warns of imminent danger – even after surgery, where the intent of the wounding is for the benefit of the person – and it signals a need for inactivity so that healing may occur (Wall, 1979). But the pain of cancer or arthritis "does not permit the organism to escape harm, nor does stillness serve to promote recovery or alleviate the pain" (Sternbach, 1989, p. 243). If and only if the suffering served a purpose could it be justified, but "whereas acute pain may promote survival, chronic pain . . . is usually destructive physically, psychologically and socially" (p. 243). With such pain come sleep disturbances, irritability, depression, inactivity, substance abuse, and disruptions of family and social life.

The meaninglessness of chronic pain is not merely noted, it is insisted upon. In *The Textbook of Pain*, the psychologist Richard A. Sternbach (1989) wrote that in some recent writings there have again been attempts to find purpose in pain: "Such writings attempt to justify God's ways to man, arguing that pain should be a part of God's ways of dealing with humans or that pain has ennobling and purifying effects on the human spirit" (p. 242). Sternbach has not found chronic pain to ennoble the spirit, and such religious views "are of little use to the investigator as clinician or researcher" (p. 242). Sternbach did not appreciate religious and philosophical justifications because chronic pain is useless and therefore meaningless. It should not be endured.

J. H. van den Berg (1974) took up Leriche's proposal that moderns suffer more from pain than our predecessors, asserting that "during this period, from 1780 until 1845, there was [an] increase of sensitivity to pain" (p. 220). He did not agree that creature comforts made nineteenth-century people more sensitive to pain; he especially disputed the notion that the introduction of aspirin at the end of the nineteenth century had this effect, because aspirin came too late to explain the change. Van den Berg's account for increased sensitivity was sociogenic. Drawing on the common observation that "pain can be made to disappear by concentrating on something" (p. 228), van den Berg related the discovery and celebration of anesthesia with changes in both social relationships and material production. Modernity is characterized by greater individual autonomy and loss of a common ground with other people. Moreover, modernity is characterized by industrial production or, in van den Berg's terms, by loss of a connection between hand and thing. Enhanced autonomy and freedom from material necessity have come at a price: "The intensity of our connection with the objects is the measure of our sensitivity to pain" (p. 228). The more connected with things we are, the less sensitive we are to pain.

This explanation sounds strange, does it not? Van den Berg was a phenomenological psychiatrist as well as a student of history. What he was reaching for with his account of increased sensitivity to pain – not an increased sensitivity in an evolutionary sense, but a sociohistorical increase – was the relationship between social relations and pain. He suggested that moderns have a changed relationship with pain because pain has been disembedded from social relationships. His basic point was that pain is more painful when we face it alone.

Algophobia: constructing acute pain

De Moulin (1974) contributed to Leriche's and van den Berg's theses. His historical review illustrated that there has never been a period in history when people did not suffer pain and seek to alleviate it – a review necessitated by extreme views of the thesis of modern pain sensitivity, which asserted the insensitivity of ancients and primitives to pain – and he concluded:

> There is no evidence that pain was once less acutely felt than in our own days. Finding no arguments that the sensitivity of our nerve system has increased in recent times, we have to attribute the rapidly dwindling readiness to accept pain to a change in our mental attitude.
>
> *(p. 569)*

De Moulin attributed the change in mental attitude to "the modern view that pain is *not* the inevitable and, in essence, irremediable result of the inherent imperfection of creation itself or of original sin, but a sign of a reparable derangement of a mechanism" (p. 569). If this is true, it means a significant change in the nature of pain. While pain in earlier times could be acute or chronic, intense, or dull, it was accepted as a matter of fact. In the words of the eighteenth-century English physician William Heberden: "I have known such a pain complained of for fifteen, sixteen, seventeen, twenty-four, and even thirty years. The more lasting of these pains are, as might be expected, moderate in degree" (1845, p. 68). Heberden, in his discussion of "dolor," acknowledged exceptions, to be sure. Some pains "are either constantly felt, or rage at certain times . . . there are others which are regularly intermittent" (p. 68). If there has been a transformation of expectations, what we should find is an expectation that pain ought to have a trajectory that leads to its cessation, either naturally or with medical aid. This expectation – this way of being toward the future – would more precisely mark the modern construction of pain. That is the contention of this chapter: Algophobia exists, and it reflects the construction of pain as naturally acute. Contrary to recent discussion on the topic, it is not chronic pain that is the modern invention or modern epidemic (although we will have to examine that assertion again later); it is acute pain, as a reality distinct from chronic pain, that is the quintessential modern phenomenon. From acute pain derives the meaninglessness of pain.

Along these lines, Witte (2014) points to the "pessimistic cultural approaches" (p. 103) to pain rooted in the notion of algophobia, which suggest that the increased sensitivity of our nervous fiber is a weakening of our moral fiber. Such attitudes contribute to mistrust of the complaints of people with chronic pain and a tendency to dismiss the reality of their suffering.

Progress, another name for algophobia

Progress, "a faith that is not recognized as such, but remains the genuine soul of the modern West and whatever comes to resemble it in the present world" (Sbert, 1992, p. 201), took form in the late eighteenth century. Progress as a secular faith refers to a belief in the inevitable perfection of the human condition. For Sbert, progress includes an implicit justification of suffering in the belief that hardships and suffering produced by economic growth are but temporary byproducts that "future perfection" (p. 195) will eliminate. While belief in progress has paled considerably in recent decades, it has had a profound influence on our attitudes toward pain, especially toward its negative status. For Vetlesen (2009), the World Health Organization's conception of health implies "the complete absence of pain and discomfort" (p. 9). Even if this eschatological fantasy shares space with very different views, it remains potent, especially in our hopes for pain reduction through technological advances.

Evidence for the belief in progress comes from Alexis de Tocqueville's *Democracy in America*, based on his journey to the United States in 1831–1832. First, he observed that in a hierarchical society, "everyone thinks that he can see the ultimate limits of human endeavor quite close in front of him" (1966, p. 419). In democratic America, these limits recede indefinitely. "Improvement" in this sense occurred in all spheres of life, but especially the material. Progress could be measured by keeping score in the pursuit of happiness. Second, the elimination of suffering was proof of progress. De Tocqueville found in America a great "taste for physical comfort." In traditional societies, he thought, both aristocrats and the lower classes did not concern themselves greatly with physical comforts: the former because their presence is assured without anxiety, the latter because "they despair of getting it and because they do not know enough about it to want it" (p. 503). But in democracies, where people see luxury as attainable, there are continually rising expectations. So whereas earlier, one could cultivate suffering, excuse the self-indulgences of those in extreme pain, and resign oneself to suffering as a poor man does to labor, now creature comforts are universally prized and tinged with anxiety. It is but a short step from this pursuit to that of new ways to alleviate pain, for no longer is the suffering of pain proof of character. Relief of discomfort and pain is liberated from the restrictions of a hierarchical social order and can be pursued in its own right, as a good in and of itself. This expectation that pain can be progressively defeated remains strong today.

In the middle of the nineteenth century, ideas of progress received support from Darwin's theory of natural selection, which "we can not fail to apply . . . to pleasure and pain," wrote Alfred Fouillée (1886, p. 682). The application: Pain is a useful adaptation if it warns us of physical danger.

> If we could imagine beings to have ever been created by any sport of Nature, whose pleasure was connected with injurious actions and their pains with useful ones, they must have died out speedily by virtue of the vice of their constitutions.
>
> *(Fouillée, 1886, p. 682)*

Pain is an "alarm bell" (Barry, 1898). In any other situation, it should be eliminated. Barry told the story of a Christian woman, Devota, who, facing surgery, felt "it a sin to evade or decline suffering," and so "she looks upon chloroform, nitrous oxide, alcohol, opium, and the rest, as unlawful drugs, means of escape which we were not intended to use." But pain, Barry replied, is not punishment; it occurs "to let us know that something has gone wrong." Its warning is "to set ourselves right, and has no value in itself," its value exhausted in its utility. He concluded, somewhat patronizingly, with Shakespeare: "'Virtue itself turns vice, being misapplied.' And so let Devota take her chloroform and thank God for sending it." Pain's utility does not extend beyond its warning of imminent physical danger.

The significance of the idea of progress for the experience of pain is twofold. First, it made an increase in material comforts an end in itself. Second, as a corollary, it made unnatural any pain that is not an alarm bell. Pain that does not warn us of harm is meaningless and intolerable. For Sarano (1970), the warning bell notion of pain limps. Pain lies. The warning often comes too late to do any good; cancer in its formative stage may produce no symptoms, and pain announces its already-advanced state. The intensity of pain does not correspond to the severity of the threat to the organism; a toothache can scream louder than a deadly infection. With progress, pain is increasingly meaningless and it must be conquered.

Expressed in an admittedly negative term, love of comfort is algophobia. The significance of algophobia is that pain is no longer necessary, and the loss of its necessity is tied here to what is called the secularization of pain.

The secularization of pain

Secularization refers to the loss of a certain type of horizon of experience and social life, the loss of the perspective of eternity when living through ordinary events. Illich (1976) and Caton (1985) argued that pain since the seventeenth century has progressively lost its transcendent meanings as a sign of evil in an imperfect world. Bourke (2014) documents these changes in detail, concluding: "Stripped of its mysticism and its function of nudging people towards more virtuous behavior, being-in-pain is emptied of a significant part of its positive value" (p. 127). Bearing with pain has ceased to be a test and a forge for spiritual purification. At its best, pain is useful biologically as a signal of danger. This transformation in the meaning of pain has rendered the experience of pain intolerable, asserted Illich and Caton. Modern anesthesia and painkilling express and reinforce this transformed attitude and did not create it. The implication of this claim is that in losing its religious significance, pain became intolerable.

The historical situation is more complex. The Christian story of the Fall and Redemption did not make pain a positive experience. Pain was one of the evils that entered the world along with death and hard work, something perhaps to be endured but not sought. Esther Cohen's (1995) study of medieval attitudes toward pain distinguished several. First is rejection, or what I have been calling algophobia: "Modern Western culture seeks as much as possible to eradicate all types of pain" (p. 51). Second is impassivity, enduring pain stoically, an attitude expressed in "no pain, no gain." Third is impassibility, "the capability of transcending pain completely" (p. 52), a gift that medieval Christians thought martyrs had been granted by God. To these, Cohen added philopassionism, which developed after the twelfth century when the humanity of the crucified Christ received attention. This new attitude expressed a desire to imitate Christ's passion: "As Christ had suffered, those who believed in him wished to suffer" (p. 59). Nevertheless, philopassionism was never the only attitude toward pain; pain was not even always cast as punishment for sin and wrongdoing, even in legal punishment. Cohen described how medieval physicians sought to alleviate pain, including the pain of surgery, and patients faced the prospect of surgery with dread and appeals to saints for succor.

Pain has and has not been secularized. Medicine has isolated it from thoughts of divine punishment. However, for many people, pain does have a spiritual meaning – as punishment, as participation in the passion of Christ, as karma, and so on. Robert Orsi (1989, 1998) shows how transcendent, religious meanings can easily rest side by side with secularized, algophobic attitudes. Catholics can ask St. Jude to intercede for them with the Almighty, take painkillers, and undergo surgery all at the same time (see Clements & Tasker, 2015). Non-Catholics make similar accommodations. The notion of secularization is a complex one. Secular and religious attitudes exist side by side in society and in individuals.

Useful pain

Illich (1976) cited Descartes' divorce of soul and body as a moment when pain ceased to be a transcendent sign: "Pain became a signal with which the body reacts in self-defense to protect its mechanical integrity" (p. 150). This is hyperbolic prose and, as we shall see, this Cartesian image of pain became dominant only at the end of the nineteenth century. However, Descartes' ability to explain body without reference to soul was significant, leading to considerations of the utility of pain.

The most prominent proponent of the utility of pain was Jeremy Bentham, and it is to his work, *An Introduction to the Principles of Morals and Legislation* (1823/1907), that we now turn. Bentham asserted that the pursuit of pleasure and the avoidance of pain are the motivating forces in human life. The sources of pleasure and pain are the natural world, political powers, other people generally, and an invisible divinity who may or may not exist. Pains resulting from natural causes are "calamities" and, metaphorically, punishments; pains caused by the law or by the neighbors are punishments. Pleasures and pains in any possible future life – the religious sanction – cannot be known by us here and now. Bentham argued for a hedonistic calculus, the measurement of the amount of pleasure or pain that can be produced – by legislation, for example.

If a definition of secularization were needed, Bentham (1823/1907) supplied one in arguing that there is no theological principle opposed to that of utility:

> [The] will of God . . . is a system which nobody ever thinks of recurring to at this time of day, for the details of political administration: and even

> before it can be applied to the details of private conduct, it is universally allowed . . . to stand in need of pretty ample interpretations.
>
> *(p. 21)*

In this instrumental approach, pain stands out, first of all, as quantifiable. The goodness or badness of an act, for an individual, can be determined by a summation of the "values of all the *pleasures* on the one side, and those of all the pains on the other" (p. 31; italics in the original). Bentham's algorithm isolated pain from the social context that hitherto had embedded it. Bentham's approach reflected and helped establish a shift in the direction of algophobia. The isolation of pain from other ends of human life and his attempt to quantify pain were significant contributions to the modern way of constructing pain.

Bentham sought to understand pleasures and pains for the purpose of conceptualizing political governance; therefore, from a critical perspective, his work is significant, because he understood that pain was a political topic. The penal system uses various forms of pain – physical, mental, and moral – to punish criminals. According to Christie (1981/2007), the penal system is largely a pain-producing enterprise. The political implications of pain extend to other areas of public life as well. Keith Wailoo (2014) has studied American legislation and legal judgments over disability benefits and found a calculus of acceptable pain during his research. What counts as pain, whose pain counts for disability assistance purposes, the meaning of suffering from pain – all are political questions in which the severity of pain only counts so much and no more. The question of the definition of pain, to which we turn in the next chapter, ramifies beyond psychological theory.

Critical perspectives

The idea of algophobia thus has its merits, but it is not by itself adequate to grasp the nature of the great divide that separates the contemporary world from 1845. To grasp the primary difference between then and now, I return to the change in existential possibilities that anesthesia and analgesics made possible. Indeed, they offered relief from pain and the temptation of drug dependence. Of course, people in pain often want some drug to kill the pain effectively. Of course, they do not want to become addicts, for that signals neediness and dependence. Of course, their painful condition means nothing except something to be overcome. For us, pain is something that can be prevented or eliminated with medication and other industrially produced comforts. This is the great divide separating us from the past.

It is not merely that we have power over pain that earlier generations did not know. In the change of life's possibilities, we have attained what earlier times sought. In this, I draw on the "theory of attainment" (Miller & Sinanan, 2014). Challenging the notion that technology alienates us from authentic life, Miller and Sinanan counter-argue that technological advances enable people to attain what they had previously only imagined or desired. Their example is the webcam, which enables people to be with others socially across great distances in ways that exceed the written letter, the telegraph, and the telephone. Applied to pain, we can say that what has been attained is the relief from pain that our ancestors desired. The term *algophobia*, while accurate, poorly and somewhat nostalgically reflects earlier centuries and their analgesic measures. Modern means of killing pain have made some earlier forms of endurance absurd and meaningless; that much is true. When something is meaningless, it is harder to endure. That is the truth of our algophobia. Pain is not dead; it is largely without – perhaps ironically – sense.

When the French Académie des Sciences debated the surgical use of ether in 1848, the physiologist François Magendie (1783–1855), who established (with Charles Bell) the distinction between sensory and motor nerves in the spinal cord, expressed grave doubts about its use. In the face of much medical opposition to his point of view, and at odds with public opinion, Magendie (quoted in Rey, 1993) expressed the concern that

> what I see most clearly in these accounts is that, with the doubtless laudable goal of operating without pain, they intoxicate their patients to the point of reducing them to what one could term the state of a cadaver which one cuts or carves with impunity and without any suffering.
>
> *(p. 163)*

The patient awake in surgery "was a source of constraint or at least of contact of obligation on the part of the surgeon" (p. 164). Magendie's views did not prevail, but he raised an important point, not for the practice of surgery, but for the existential changes occurring at the time. The anatomical image of the body was socially instituted with anesthesia. The person's "abandoned body" was at the disposal of the surgeon for the occasion of surgery. One of the implications of this shift to the medical gaze and the objectified body as a social institution was that the cadaver became the guide to the flesh of the living (see Bishop, 2011). A second implication was that pain would have to be located in the cadaver in order to be "real pain." What is also the case is that, unlike the hopes of someone like Silas Weir Mitchell and his poem "The Birth and Death of Pain," pain had not died, not even when reduced to something like sensory pain. To these topics we now turn.

References

Acker, C. J. (1995). From all-purpose anodyne to marker of deviance: Physicians' attitudes toward opiates from 1890 to 1940. In R. Porter & M. Teich (Eds.), *Drugs and narcotics in history* (pp. 114–132). Cambridge, England: Cambridge University Press.

Altick, R. D. (1997). *Punch: The lively youth of a British institution, 1841–1851*. Columbus: Ohio State University Press.

Armstrong, T. (2012). *The logic of slavery: Debt, technology, and pain in American literature*. Cambridge, England: Cambridge University Press.

Bain, A. (1859). *The emotions and the will*. London, England: Parker.

Barry, W. (1898). The ethics of pain. *Public Opinion, 25*(26), 823.

Bentham, J. (1907). *An introduction to the principles of morals and legislation*. Oxford, England: Clarendon Press. (Original work published 1823)

Bishop, J. P. (2011). *The anticipatory corpse: Medicine, power, and the care of the dying*. Notre Dame, IN: University of Notre Dame Press.

The blessing of ether. (1847). *Punch, 12*, 141.

The blessings of chloroform. (1848). *Punch, 13*, 232.

Bonica, J. J. (1953). *The management of pain*. Philadelphia, PA: Lea & Febiger.

Bonner, T. N. (1995). *Becoming a physician: Medical education in Great Britain, France, Germany, and the United States, 1750–1945*. Oxford, England: Oxford University Press.

Bourke, J. (2014). *The story of pain: From prayer to painkillers*. Oxford, England: Oxford University Press. http://dx.doi.org/10.14296/RiH/2014/1656

Buytendijk, F.J.J. (1962). *Pain: Its modes and functions* (E. O'Shiel, Trans.). Chicago, IL: University of Chicago Press.

Caton, D. (1985). The secularization of pain. *Anesthesiology, 62*, 493–501.

Chisholm, J. J. (1861). *A manual of military surgery for the use of surgeons in the Confederate States Army*. Charleston, SC: Evans & Cogswell.

Chloroform. (1848, January 28). *Vermont Phoenix*, p. 3. Retrieved from http://chroniclingamerica.loc.gov/

Chloroform. (1848, February 8). *New York Daily Tribune*, p. 4. Retrieved from http://chroniclingamerica.loc.gov/

Christie, N. (2007). *Limits to pain: The role of punishment in penal policy*. Eugene, OR: Wipf & Stock. (Original work published 1981)

Clements, F., & Tasker, F. (2015). Living through the Paschal Mystery: Surviving cancer narratives told by older Roman Catholic women. *Journal of Religion, Spirituality & Aging, 27*(1), 48–66. http://dx.doi.org/10.1080/15528030.2014.943452

Cohen, E. (1995). Towards a history of European physical sensibility: Pain in the later Middle Ages. *Science in Context, 8*, 47–74.

De Moulin, D. (1974). A historical-phenomenological study of bodily pain in Western man. *Bulletin of the History of Medicine, 48*, 540–570.

De Tocqueville, A. (1966). *Democracy in America* (J. P. Mayer & M. Lerner, Eds.; G. Lawrence, Trans.). New York, NY: Harper & Row.

Dormandy, T. (2006). *The worst of evils: The fight against pain*. New Haven, CT: Yale University Press.

Duden, B. (1991). *The woman beneath the skin: A doctor's patients in eighteenth-century Germany* (T. Dunlap, Trans.). Cambridge, MA: Harvard University Press.

Foucault, M. (1973). *The birth of the clinic* (A.M.S. Smith, Trans.). New York, NY: Vintage Books.

Fouillée, A. (1886). The nature of pleasure and pain. *Popular Science Monthly, 29*, 681–693.

Halttunen, K. (1995). Humanitarianism and the pornography of pain in Anglo-American culture. *American Historical Review, 100*, 303–334. http://dx.doi.org/10.2307/2169001

Heberden, W. (1845). *Commentaries on the history and cure of diseases*. Philadelphia, PA: Barrington & Haswell.

Hulkower, R. (2011). From sacrilege to privilege: The tale of body procurement for anatomical dissection in the United States. *The Einstein Journal of Biology and Medicine, 27*(1), 23–26.

Illich, I. (1976). *Medical nemesis: The expropriation of health*. New York, NY: Pantheon.

Illich, I. (2005). *Rivers north of the future: The testimony of Ivan Illich as told to David Cayley*. Toronto, ON, Canada: Anansi Press.

Inhalation of ethereal vapor. (1847, January 7). *Voice of Freedom*, p. 1. Retrieved from http://chroniclingamerica.loc.gov/

Kimball, H. (1846). Morton's lethêon. In *Circular: Morton's Lethêon* (pp. 22–25). Boston, MA: Bridgham. Retrieved from https://archive.org/details/0312644.nlm.nih.gov

Leriche, R. (1939). *The surgery of pain* (A. Young, Trans.). Baltimore, MD: Williams & Wilkins.

The meaning of pain. (1906). *The Living Age*, 7th Series, 30, *248*(3219), 699–701.

Miller, D., & Sinanan, J. (2014). *Webcam*. Cambridge, England: Polity Press.

Mitchell, S. W. (1900). The birth and death of pain. In *The wager and other poems* (pp. 15–19). New York, NY: Century.

Morris, D. (1991). *The culture of pain*. Berkeley: University of California Press.

Morrison, L. A., & Sharples, S. P. (1897). *History of the Kimball family in America, from 1634 to 1897* (Vol. 2). Boston, MA: Damrell & Upham. Retrieved from https://archive.org/details/historyofkimball02byumorr

Musto, D. F. (1999). *The American disease: Origins of narcotic control*. New York, NY: Oxford University Press.

The new discovery in surgery. (1847). *Punch, 12*, 22.

Orsi, R. (1989). The cult of the saints and the reimagination of the space and time of sickness in twentieth-century American Catholicism. *Medicine & Literature, 8*, 66–73.

Orsi, R. (1998). *Thank you, Saint Jude: Women's devotion to the patron saint of hopeless causes*. New Haven, CT: Yale University Press.

Osler, W. (1929). *Bibliotheca Osleriana: A catalogue of books illustrating the history of medicine and science*. Oxford, England: Clarendon.

Painless operation. (1847). *Punch, 12*, 81.

Papper, E. M. (1995). *Romance, poetry, and surgical sleep: Literature influences medicine*. Westport, CT: Greenwood.

Pernick, M. S. (1985). *A calculus of suffering: Pain, professionalism, and anesthesia in nineteenth-century America*. New York, NY: Columbia University Press.

Reiser, S. J. (1978). *Medicine and the reign of technology*. Cambridge, England: Cambridge University Press.

Rey, R. (1993). *The history of pain* (L. E. Wallace, J. A. Cadden, & S. W. Cadden, Trans.). Cambridge, MA: Harvard University Press.

Richardson, B. W. (1897). *Vita medica: Chapters of medical life and work*. London, England: Longmans, Green.

Romanyshyn, R. (1989). *Technology as symptom and dream*. New York, NY: Routledge.

Sarano, J. (1970). *The hidden face of pain* (D. Pardee, Trans.). Valley Forge, PA: Judson Press.

Sbert, J. M. (1992). Progress. In W. Sachs (Ed.), *The development dictionary* (pp. 192–205). London, England: Zed.

Schiller, F. (1990). The history of algology, algotherapy, and the role of inhibition. *Pubbicazioni della Stazione Zoologica di Napoli, Section II: History and Philosophy of the Life Sciences, 12*, 27–50.

Sonnedecker, G. (1976). *Kremers and Urdang's history of pharmacy* (4th ed.). Philadelphia, PA: Lippincott.

Stanley, P. (2003). *For fear of pain: British surgery, 1790–1850*. Amsterdam, Netherlands: Rodopi.

Stelmackowich, C. (2012). The instructive corpse: Dissection, anatomical specimens, and illustration in early nineteenth-century medical education. *Spontaneous Generations: A Journal for the History and Philosophy of Science, 6*(1), 50–64.

Sternbach, R. A. (1989). Acute versus chronic pain. In P. D. Wall & R. Melzack (Eds.), *Textbook of pain* (2nd ed., pp. 242–246). Edinburgh, Scotland: Churchill Livingston.

van den Berg, J. H. (1972). *A different existence: Principles of phenomenological psychopathology*. Pittsburgh, PA: Duquesne University Press.

van den Berg, J. H. (1974). *Divided existence and complex society.* Pittsburgh, PA: Duquesne University Press.

Vetlesen, A. J. (2009). *A philosophy of pain.* London, England: Reaktion Books.

Wailoo, K. (2014). *Pain: A political history.* Baltimore, MD: Johns Hopkins University Press.

Wall, P. D. (1979). On the relation of injury to pain. *Pain, 6*, 253–264.

Wallis, P. (2004). Richardson, Sir Benjamin Ward (1828–1896). Retrieved from www.oxforddnb.com/view/article/23544

Witte, W. (2014). The emergence of chronic pain: Phantom limbs, subjective experience and pain management in post-war West Germany. In R. Boddice (Ed.), *Pain and emotion in modern history* (pp. 90–110). New York, NY: Palgrave Macmillan.

Wonderful effects of ether in case of scolding wife. (1847). *Punch, 12*, 60.

2

CONSTRUCTING REAL PAIN

The understanding of pain that came to dominate by the end of the nineteenth century has been called the "sensation theory" of pain. According to this theory, pain, like touch or vision, originates in a stimulation of a sensory nerve, which is transmitted to the brain and registered as a sensation. Emotional, cognitive, and motivational factors then follow. Guiding medical intervention for most of the following century, the sensation theory was an innovative approach to the nature of pain. Its development was contingent upon knowledge gained of the body from anatomy and physiology, which became the basis of medical practice in the nineteenth century. In particular, it has its roots in the study of the nervous system. The new theories of pain spatialized it; that is, pain became something that could be visualized in the body. This construction of pain promised new control over pain, because pain could be located. Acceptance of the sensation theory meant the displacement of the then-dominant conception of pain as a quality of consciousness coupled with pleasure. To grasp the spatialization of pain, a brief look at nineteenth-century interest in the spinal cord is in order.

Locating pain in the spinal cord and nerves

Sir Charles Bell, the British physiologist, was one recipient of dead bodies stolen from the grave. Bell's work, distinguishing the functions of the anterior and posterior roots of the spinal cord, significantly affected the understanding of pain, leading to the sensation theory. Contemporary research by François Magendie led to the "Bell–Magendie law," which stated that the posterior roots transmit sensory impulses and the anterior roots transmit motor impulses. In 1832, Marshall Hall established the spinal reflex arc, which connects sensory and motor action in the cord. Schiller (1990) concluded that "the Cartesian approach [in the work of Bell, Magendie, and Hall] had caused a revaluation: away from [pain's] mental and moral aspects pain became a useful factor in the working of the biological machine" (p. 37). This conception is Cartesian because the nerve pathway connected nerve action at the periphery of the body to the brain; pain is felt when the signal reaches the brain. In Descartes, that was where the soul resided and felt the impulse as pain.

Johannes Müller established that "each sense is related to its own specific anatomical pattern of nerve fibres" (Keele, 1957, p. 109), the law of specific nerve energy, a teaching that grounded subsequent physiological analysis of sensation. Müller's results "represent a systematic expression of the observations of Bell and his followers up to the middle of the century, and constitute the basis upon which a large part of the later work was founded" (p. 108). The nineteenth century saw much research on sensory and motor pathways in the nervous system (Finger, 1994). By the late 1860s, investigations showed that there were "different sensory modes following different paths in the spinal cord" (Keele, 1957, p. 113). For pain to be received as a sensation, receptors in the periphery needed to be identified and, based on research into other cutaneous sensory areas of the skin (Norrsell, Finger, & Lajonchere, 1999), Max von Frey in 1894 claimed to have found nerve endings in the skin that transmitted pain signals. Von Frey's "surprisingly popular theory" was "immediately challenged by anatomists" (Norrsell, Finger, & Lajonchere, 1999, p. 463). Debates over pain nerves continued for decades, even as the sensation theory took root in medicine and psychology.

The sensation theory became the dominant way in which to understand pain in medicine in the first half of the twentieth century, despite strong arguments against it by other physiological investigators (Bonica, 1990, p. 8). Keele (1957), writing triumphantly in the middle of the century, proclaimed that "it was due to von Frey, more than anyone else, that at the beginning of the twentieth century the concept of a rigid neural architecture subserving pain took firm root, and has flourished ever since" (p. 132). Its main competitor in the first half of the twentieth century was the pattern theory, which states that "a specific sensation results when the brain receives from the skin impulses which make up a characteristic pattern, built up from both spatial and temporal components" (p. 134). For both theories, pain is a sensation. A retrospective assessment concludes:

> As for pain, the most puzzling of the skin senses, most researchers now agree that there are special receptors to warn against tissue damage – the so-called nociceptors. Threshold activation of nociceptors, however, may be insufficient to cause a pain sensation. Further it has been shown that pain can be evoked without activating these nociceptors.
>
> *(Norrsell et al., 1999, p. 464)*

Bonica (1952) captured the received view of pain: "Pain involves perception of noxious impulses and a reaction thereto" (p. 1582). In 1950, pain was still viewed as a sensation along the lines of vision and touch. While the sensation theory could not account for all pain phenomena (nor could the pattern theory), in medical textbooks, the sensation theory dominated (Bonica, 1990, p. 8; Schiller, 1990). Viewing pain as fundamentally a sensation inscribed it in the anatomical image of the body. The sensation theory had great promise for the treatment of pain. However, before the identification of pain with sensation achieved dominance in psychology, it was fiercely debated.

Pain as quality, pain as sensation

Morris (1991) observes that "we live in an era when many people believe – as a basic, unexamined foundation of thought – that pain comes divided into separate types: physical and mental" (p. 9), in large part because of the "medical myth" (p. 4) that pain is a sensation. We turn now to a controversy over this myth at a time when it was becoming dominant in psychology and medicine.

At the end of the nineteenth century, psychologists debated the nature of pain (Dallenbach, 1939). Some supported the sensation theory; others paired pleasure with pain and viewed them both as qualities (*qualês*) of mental states. The quality theory of pain had Henry Rutgers Marshall as its leading proponent. An examination of this debate sheds light on which possibilities for the experience and treatment of pain were being opened and closed at the turn of the new century.

That a neurological conception of pain should have superseded a psychological one is not surprising. The debate took place in the wake of the acceptance of surgical anesthesia, the proliferation of analgesics, and the proclaimed "death of pain," after all. Physiology was a leading science of the day, promising a scientific understanding of vital activities, and the life sciences were seen to have bearing on the significance of mental life, culture, religion, and human nature generally. In psychology proper, the "new psychology" was largely physiological in orientation, drawing on work such as that of Helmholtz and Fechner on the nervous system. If psychology was to become truly scientific, surely extensions of this neurological perspective were in order. For William James (1892), for example, understanding the neurological basis of mental life was essential if psychology were to become a natural science.

Classifying mental life

The exchanges to which Marshall (1889) first contributed his particular view of pleasure and pain were not initially about pain nerves. They concerned the conceptual categories appropriate for mental life, the analysis of which was being pursued by philosophical psychologists, including Alexander Bain, James Ward, and F. H. Bradley. The conversation had been going on for a long time; we pick it up with Ward (1887), who claimed that there was much conceptual confusion in psychology regarding basic terms, a point made by other leading figures, although "they agreed that psychology has its own subject-matter and cannot be studied as a function of nervous processes" (Smith, 2013, p. 78). Ward noted ambiguities in Bain's use of "feeling," which could mean sensations and emotions (F_1) on the one hand and pleasures, pains, and excited states (F_2) on the other hand. For Ward, pleasure and pain were not sensations because they had no specific sense organ as do the senses, and they were not emotions; of course, there were pleasurable and painful sensations and emotions. Ward concluded that F_1 were presentations – that is, states of consciousness that presented some content – e.g., a color. For Ward, F_2 were subjective states – feelings – that result from presentations: *How do you feel about that color?* Pleasure and pain did not refer to objects and thus were not presentations. Bradley (1887) disagreed, arguing that pleasure and pain were indeed presentations because they have objects: the pleasant and the painful. Bain (1887) acknowledged the "unavoidable vagueness of subjective phenomena" (p. 576), arguing that feelings included more than pleasure and pain; they also referred to "neutral modes" of excitement, such as those that accompany "the din of a London street" (p. 577). Feelings could be pleasurable or painful, but they might be neither. They were states of "conscious intensity" (p. 578), the opposite of repose. Like Ward, for Bain, feelings were the subjective side of mental life.

This debate continued without resolution. Bradley (1888) contended that pleasure and pain, as presentations, were initially neither subjective nor objective; only as experience becomes elaborated does this distinction take place. He remarked, however, that "the action of pain is to excite change away from what is painful" (p. 12), tying feelings to action. Restlessness is the "chief effect of pain" (p. 14), an important point to which we shall return in discussing the phenomenology of pain.

Marshall on pleasure and pain

When Marshall (1889) contributed to the conversation, he proposed a classification of pleasure and pain. He disputed the position of Ward and Bain that pleasure and pain were feelings. Instead, he claimed that pleasure and pain were qualities of presentations. He disagreed with the common-sense view that "naturally thinks of Pain as a Sensation and of Pleasure as an Emotion" (p. 517). For Marshall, the primary quality at issue was pleasure-pain, what he also called the algedonic quality. Every state of consciousness must be painful, pleasurable, or indifferent (as a transition between the two poles). By quality, Marshall meant a differentiation of a mental state. Pleasure-pain belonged to the "primary *quales* which affect *all* presentation, however wide, however narrow" (p. 527; italics in the original). Pleasure-pain was but one general quality of relation that Marshall claimed belongs to all presentations. Other general qualities were intensity, manifoldness (differentiation of parts), realness, and time. Marshall distinguished between these general qualities and what he called "special qualities," such as color or tone, that characterize presentations such as sensations. The algedonic quality affected every element within the complex of a conscious moment, such that the total experience could be one of mixed feeling. For Marshall, there were pleasurable and painful sensations and emotions, but pleasure and pain were neither. While acknowledging differences among painful experiences, for Marshall the pain of physically and mentally painful states was the same *qualê* – pain: "I do not consider this separation of physical from other pleasures and pains fundamentally important" (1909b, p. 102). In part, this position stemmed from his insistence that pleasure and pain are aspects of the same *qualê*: "If we separate *schmerz* [physical pain] from *unlust* [disagreeableness], we should in like manner separate sense pleasures from other pleasures" (1909b, p. 101). We "tend to emphasize pain as sensation" (p. 101), Marshall reasoned, because tissue damage commonly produced physical pain. Pleasures are not necessarily derived from analogous conditions, and so they tend to be seen more in emotional than sensory terms. In this classification of conscious experience, Marshall was following the lead of earlier empiricist thinkers, although some of the details were his own. Marshall developed his theory of pain in a series of essays (1889, 1891a, 1891b, 1892, 1894a, 1895a, 1895b, 1909a) and in a book (1894b).

At stake was what we understand pain – and pleasure – to be. Marshall (1894b) defined them broadly, following "common sense" (p. 3), for which there are many types of pains and pleasures, some of the flesh and some of the mind, especially the aesthetic. In making these distinctions, he was in line with John Stuart Mill, who had asserted the "superiority of mental over bodily pleasures" (Mill, 1863, p. 11). Marshall similarly differentiated pleasures and pains: "Intellectual pleasures and pains are no meaningless terms; they are as full of actual import as are the phrases sensational and emotional pleasures and pains" (1894b, pp. 35–36). To this list of types of pains, others added moral pain, which "is just as real as physical pain" (Cecil, 1910, p. 20). This was an expansive conception of pain that Marshall and others defended, and it reflected common-sense understandings.

Physiological correlates of pleasure and pain

Pleasure and pain are mental contents of some sort, or so these psychological theorists taught. Yet they must have some bodily cause or correlate. Marshall (1891a, 1891b) reviewed thinking on this topic from the Greeks to his day and offered his own theory. Not holding that pleasure or pain are sensations, he did not hypothesize specific nerves mediating them. Marshall (1891b) looked to the organism as a whole, and he concluded that "Pleasure is produced by the use of stored force in the organ determining the [mental] content; and Pain is determined by the reception of a stimulus to which the organ is incapable of reacting completely" (p. 471). This proposal was modern in the sense that it invoked energetic considerations, which figured prominently in the biology of the time (Rabinbach, 1990).

To this nutrition-based theory of the algedonic quality Marshall later added a "neururgic" account, according to which pleasure and pain "relate respectively to the efficiency and inefficiency of the *neural elements* whose activity corresponds with the pleasant or painful presentations" (1909b, p. 251; italics in the original). Marshall's physiological theory resembled psychodynamic thinking, for it emphasized the energetic character of pain and pleasure: "When the activity of the nerve that is the correlate of the experienced mental item involves the use of surplus stored energy, this mental item is characterized by *pleasure*" (1920, p. 137; italics in the original), with pain defined as the correlate of a deficit of energy. Speculations about mental energy abounded at the time in the psychologies of Janet, Freud, Jung, and others from the same period.

Marshall's critics found his understanding of pain wanting. William James (1894) pointed out that "at present, while professing to be physiological, the law is really, they will say, quite 'transcendental' " (p. 50). Lightner Witmer (1894) called the nutritional basis of pleasure and pain not in keeping with "the method of scientific physiology" (p. 227) and stated that the *qualê* "theory is a bit of psychological drift wood that has been thrown before the feet of the modern psychologist by the waves of past speculation" (p. 210).

Bain (1892) found Marshall's theory adequate for certain pleasures and pains – namely, active use of the muscles (pleasurable) and muscular fatigue (painful). Other pains, such as that accompanying bitter taste, he found less explained by Marshall's theory, and although it points in the right direction, there were too many "anomalies and exceptions" (p. 185) for it to hold generally. This search for a bodily basis of pleasure and pain changed, however, as neurological considerations came to the fore. Marshall's position, equating pleasure with reserve force and pain with insufficient power, owed much to earlier nineteenth-century understandings of nerve force.

Marshall never abandoned his proposed physiological basis of pain-pleasure. Some psychologists took it seriously. George Frederick Stout (1899) incorporated it into his own hypothetical accounts of the biological basis of pleasure and pain. He suggested

> that when wear outruns repair the experience is displeasing, and that when repair outruns wear the experience is pleasing. On this view it is difficult to account for the fact that pleasures may be exhausting, and that when they are long-continued, they diminish, and pass into displeasure.
>
> *(p. 236)*

He discussed Marshall's views, objecting that the theory did not account for all pleasures and pains. For one thing, it cannot account for individual differences in pleasures and pains. Second, "surplus energy" is not defined by the theory. Stout concluded by observing "how speculative and insecure, in the present state of our knowledge, hypotheses of this kind are" (p. 240).

The sensation theory: a neurological interpretation of pain and pleasure

The second half of the nineteenth century saw extensive neurological and psychophysical research on the senses. By the end of the century, investigations of the cutaneous senses were under way, with contributions from researchers such as Blix, Goldscheider, Donaldson, and von Frey. While that research sailed along unimpeded by Marshall's objections, there was a series of exchanges on the topic that highlight what was at stake for an understanding of pain. Herbert Nichols, then a psychologist at Harvard, presented a version of the sensation theory of pleasure and pain, partly in reply to Marshall, and to which Marshall responded. Nichols (1892a) took exception to the long-held view that pleasure and pain were opposites. Nichols changed the hermeneutic principles for understanding pleasure and pain, and that turn is more significant than his theory. For Nichols, the ground of understanding was "the modern notions of strict correspondence between all psychic phenomena and their neural basis" (p. 405). Further, if pleasure and pain appear as psychic phenomena, they must be sensations, "as fundamental elements of mind" (p. 404). It is important to stress that the debates between Marshall and his contemporaries had to do with their starting point: Marshall began with an analysis of consciousness, and Nichols began with a search for the neural correlates of consciousness.

Nichols (1892a) founded his approach in the doctrine of specific nerve energy; if there is a sensation, then there is a nerve that causes it. He cited the work of Goldscheider, who reported "having discovered and positively demonstrated isolated specific pain nerves" (p. 406). He drew on experiential evidence in support of this view:

> With a pin I touch certain points on the back of my hand in the slightest possible manner. Long after the visible touch is made, a sharp definite pain comes swelling in, out of all proportion to the pin-touch and entirely unaccompanied with any other resulting sensation.
>
> *(p. 405)*

At no time in this little experiment did the pain change and become pleasure. He also cited evidence from the administration of chloroform, cocaine, and ice: Pain sensations can disappear separately from other sensory experiences. Nichols also proposed that pleasure nerves must exist, and he made an argument on evolutionary ground that pleasure, which incites movement toward a stimulus, must have been the primary sense that organisms possess, given its strong connections with food and sex. The more complex pleasures of higher organisms, he proposed, are based on associative learning. In extending this evolutionary argument, Nichols (1892b) made the argument that pain functions as a warning system. Since pain inspires action to reduce pain, "our pains must be essentially beneficial, in order to have been so fundamentally and widely wrought up into our developed organism. Had their general function been detrimental, it would have become eliminated" (p. 523). In this way, Nichols fleshed out neurologically the construction of pain as essentially acute pain, the prototype of pain.

Marshall (1892) acknowledged that Nichols made the case for the sensation theory. One important point in Marshall's reply was that the field of consciousness is a complex unity: "The mind acts as a totality, and the relations between its special partial activities must be embodied in consciousness even though the functioning of no special distinct organ be coincident with the grasp by us of these relations" (p. 641) – that is, there is no one-to-one correlation between a state of consciousness and the underlying neural activity. As far as Goldscheider's claim to have discovered pain nerves, in addition to citing authorities who dispute the claim – Blix, Wundt, and Ladd – Marshall suggested that the so-called pain nerves could be artifacts of the experiment in which they were allegedly isolated (p. 631). He concluded by asserting that introspection, or appeal to first-person experience, is the ultimate authority for psychological investigations. If Nichols's argument had turned that upside down, Marshall sought to upright it.

Nichols (1896) insisted upon a correlation between pain and nerve action: "That specific nerves of pain have at last been established with a certainty fully equal to that for any of the other dermal nerves is an event, for psychology, of the first magnitude" (p. 309). He cited the experimental work of Henry Head, which showed that "the skin of the body is divided into definitive zones of nerve-supply for pain" (p. 309). Nichols concluded by saying that von Frey's evidence, together with Head's, should "convert the most fastidious from the time-honored superstitions" (p. 313). George Santayana (1894) summarized the main thrust of the critics: "Introspection cannot distinguish perceptions from the qualities of perceptions. . . . The question becomes real and not verbal only in the field of physiology" (p. 413).

Bain (1892) sided with Marshall in keeping pleasure bound with pain and in not defining either as a simple sensation. He noted the evidence of experience, including that of aesthetic and ethical pleasures and pains. Bain stated that "a theory of pleasure and pain is wanting if it does not somehow introduce us to the very great variety of modes of both the one and the other" (p. 187). Marshall's theory was an advance, but Bain found it lacking in some fundamental respects, not only for the simpler pleasures and pains but also for "the intense enjoyments and severe pains allied with the Amicable and the Malevolent modes" (p. 187) of the emotions.

A key point in these exchanges had to do with the basis for interpretation. Marshall, as we have seen, argued that introspection was its ground. For others, such as Witmer, who strenuously defended the natural scientific approach in psychology, physiology was also a ground for understanding mental life. On this basis, Witmer took issue with Marshall's physiological speculations, claiming that the existence of pain nerves was compatible with introspective analysis. A purely introspective psychological analysis was not immune from correction by physiology: "Psychology never ceased to consider all sensations arising from stimulation of the skin as one group, namely, the so called sensations of feeling, until histology revealed disparate peripheral terminals" (Witmer, 1894, p. 214). In this article, Witmer did not abandon introspection as a legitimate method in psychology, and he presented psychological and physiological investigations as complementary. Nevertheless, his principal objection to Marshall's *qualê* theory was that, on its basis, "no satisfactory physiological explanation of pleasure and pain is possible" (p. 227).

Witmer (1894) objected to neurologists taking Marshall seriously. Indeed, Charles L. Dana, a leading neurologist, did. While he seemed to assume that

Marshall's views represented a majority of psychologists – a point that Witmer sought to correct – Dana observed that pain "is a subjective or common sensation," unlike touch, which "is objective" ("Syringo-Myelia," 1894, p. 70). He concluded that "pain is much more closely allied to hunger than it is to touch. Pain is not a special sensation, but a modification of it" (p. 70). It made no sense to him, therefore, to look for pain tracts in the spinal cord. Another neurologist, Joseph Collins (1894), reviewed Marshall's (1894b) book favorably, but he took issue with Marshall's dismissal of the existence of pain nerves and a pain center in the brain. Physiological studies, pathological data, and weaknesses of the *qualê* theory combined suggested to Collins that pain was indeed a sensation. As to Marshall's physiological theory, Collins thought that it did not have "any *raison d'être*" (p. 276).

The professional environments of psychologists debating pain

The American psychologists who supported the sensation theory were proponents of experimental psychology. Witmer, after studies with Wundt, became director of the laboratory established by James McKeen Cattell at the University of Pennsylvania in 1892. Anna Jane McKeag, a student of Witmer's, conducted experimental studies on pain for her dissertation (McKeag, 1902). Nichols taught psychology at both Harvard and Johns Hopkins in the 1890s after earning a Ph.D. at Clark under Stanley Hall in 1891 (Dallenbach, 1937). Charles A. Strong taught at the University of Chicago (1892–1895), where he opened the first experimental psychology laboratory (Garvey, 1929), and at Columbia (1896–1913). Other experimental psychologists contributed to the establishment of the sensation theory of pain. George Washington Andrew Luckey (1895) wrote an important review of the scientific literature on pain. Edgar A. Singer (1897) conducted experimental studies at the Harvard Psychological Laboratory using von Frey's and Goldscheider's methods. Harold Griffing (1897), at Columbia University, reviewed a monograph of von Frey and conducted (Griffing, 1896) studies of individual differences in pain sensitivity using an algometer designed by Cattell, observing in conclusion that "not knowing the path of the current in the body, we have no right to assume any special physiological or psychological basis for the data obtained from introspection" (p. 415). Dallenbach (1939) – no neutral observer and a student of Titchener, he conducted related studies – wrote that "psychologists moved over to the sensory view almost in a body. Here was something definite to teach, and textbooks changed over night" (p. 340) after physiological studies described "pain nerves." Narrow fibers conveyed pain and helped convey psychology into the modern world of the natural sciences.

These psychologists worked at modern research universities. The American university scene in the 1890s "favored specialization" (Danziger, 1990, p. 40), and in psychology that meant physiological psychology. As Wolfe (1895) declared, "the rapid development of laboratories for the study of Physiological and Experimental Psychology has silenced the chief objections to such methods of investigating the facts of mind" (p. 382).

The quality theorists, also teachers for the most part, maintained strong philosophical interests. However, Marshall was an architect and taught only occasionally. An early member of the American Psychological Association, becoming its president in 1907, he objected to the growing preoccupation with methodology in psychology. Marshall championed introspection, but he never – unlike Titchener – attempted to make it into an experimental technique. For Marshall, introspection was a mode of educated self-consciousness. Marshall lacked an institutional setting that would enable his approach and his theories to propagate, whatever their intrinsic merits. Method was coming to dominate psychological praxis, and the research-oriented university setting was the ground on which natural scientific psychology grew.

As Danziger (1996) argues, "scientific discourse [is] . . . a socially embedded dialogue between theory and practice" (p. 18), with practice often dictating theory rather than vice versa (p. 17). Methodological considerations differentiated the sensation and the quality theories of pain, holding sway in the former, while in the latter having a subsidiary place. The discourse on method among the quality theorists was more in the tradition of Descartes and Locke: systematic reflection on the representations in the mind. The centrality of method for the sensation theorists stemmed from their interests in the scientific status of psychology. Discord over the importance of methodology differentiated the two discourses. The differing emphasis on objective methodologies interacted with the psychological practices of the psychologists and their institutional settings. The sensation theorists demanded physiological and psychophysical evidence, with devices such as the algometer inscribing the distinctions that physiology described onto experimental subjects and students. This experimentally based discourse and praxis functioned, moreover, to legitimate psychological expertise, and it promised, in the hands of Witmer and others, practical applications. Marshall's discourse, on the other hand, secured neither disciplinary identity nor institutional setting, since it could be accomplished outside the laboratory and the university.

Constructing real pain

Marshall's broad conception of pain provoked comment. James (1894) queried:

> Are the various forms of displeasure of which we are susceptible, rightly to be gathered up under the single name of "pain"? . . . Might not "pain" *par excellence* . . . and nausea also, well be energies of specific nerves, while the milder and less localized displeasures might be such "*qualês*" as Mr. Marshall contends for?
>
> *(p. 50)*

Witmer (1894) also challenged the assumption that the painful and the disagreeable were identical phenomena and also the link Marshall supposed between pain and pleasure.

The distinction between pain and displeasure was still being argued some years later. Mary Calkins (1916) remarked that "it is . . . less easy to realize that painfulness is quite distinct also from disagreeableness or unpleasantness. Half the experiences which we ordinarily call 'painful' are probably merely unpleasant" (p. 71). The confusion arises in part because "painful things are also unpleasant" (p. 72). But the argument turned on the "fact" that "there is probably only a single quality of pain-sensation," even though "at first thought, this statement may seem to contradict our ordinary experience" (p. 72). In ordinary experience, we rarely have pain sensations alone. In reply to these criticisms, Marshall (1920) continued to assert the broad usage of the word *pain* because it accords with common experience. The common man, he wrote, "looks upon pain as clearly marked and emphatic disagreeableness; or, to put it in the obverse way, he looks upon disagreeableness as diffused and moderate pain" (p. 136, unnumbered footnote).

Luckey's (1895) review of the debate began with the uncertainties:

> Whether it [pain] is of physiological or psychological origin; whether it is mediated by specific nerves, or by any or all sensory nerves; whether pain is to be considered as a *quale* of a sensation, a separate, coördinate sensation, or only an intense degree of a sensation; – for on all these points our knowledge of pain is far from satisfactory.
>
> *(p. 108)*

For Luckey, Marshall's *qualê* theory was wanting; he noted studies by Schiff that found separate pathways in the spinal cord for pain and other haptic feelings (p. 112). For the variation of the sensation theory that postulated specific pain nerves, Luckey discussed von Frey's experiments and Nichols's theory. Von Frey had used mechanical and electrical stimulation to provoke painful feelings on the skin and found areas of the skin that yielded pain points but no touch points, and vice versa. However, Luckey "remained doubtful whether such nerves exist" (p. 116). He favored Goldscheider's alternative for the sensation theory – the view that intensity of stimulation and summation of nerve impulses determine pain sensations. Goldscheider tied what Luckey called "real pain" to "pressure nerves and the nerves of common feeling. . . . Sensations of other sense nerves may be unpleasant, but not really painful" (in Luckey, p. 120). For Goldscheider, "pain is due to an increasing sensitiveness in the spinal ganglion cells" (in Luckey, p. 121). Pain is "a new element added to other sensations" (Luckey, p. 121). Rather than seeing pain as itself a sensation, Luckey suggested that it is "an intensive degree of a sensation" (p. 121). With Goldscheider, Luckey concluded by identifying something he explicitly called "real pain" (p. 123).

The adjective *real* is a particular type of qualifier, as Hacking (1995) points out, as it implies something else that is not real. For Marshall, intellectual and aesthetic pains were pains; for the position that Luckey articulated, following neurological investigations, they were not real or really pains. What did this do to the "experience" of pain?

What we see in the establishment of the sensation theory is a redefinition of the meaning of experience. The experimental situation framed the appearance of a "sensation." The experimental method produced the sensation of pain in the experimental subject. The experiment taught psychologists what a sensation was. Titchener (1901) instructed students to distinguish between sensations produced by a bristle and a needle:

> The sensations of *pain* are very different from either the temperature or the pressure sensations. They are minutely fine, wirelike, then; much livelier and more thrill-like than the pressure sensations. . . . The pain sensations have no bigness at all.
>
> *(p. 95)*

Contemporaries were aware of this social construction of sensations; McKeag (1902) observed that "the subject's apperception-mass is . . . an important factor in the production of the judgment" (pp. 3–4). Her comment related to one of her subjects, who differentiated pain from pressure on the basis of prior knowledge of Goldscheider's terminology (p. 7). Luckey (1895) raised the objection, germane to this point, of an arbitrary construction of sensations:

> A touch with the point of a needle . . . will often produce, first, a sensation of touch, and, after a second, another distinct, long-continued sensation of intense itching; on stronger stimulation, there may be first touch and pain, followed by a long-continued sensation of itching. Shall we, therefore, assume itching nerves and itching points?
>
> *(p. 117)*

Experimental introspection was a complex set of practices (Danziger, 1980; Wozniak, 1993) that isolated an element from the "total experience" (McKeag, 1902, p. 14), an element that could be identified as distinct, even if it never appeared by itself outside the laboratory. A dialectic of theory and praxis established an object – "pain as a sensation" – in the new experimental and academic settings.

A decisive point was made by Strong (1896), whose analysis helped establish a distinction between pain and displeasure: "I propose, therefore, to take up the experience of cutaneous pain, and to look at it first from the neurological and afterwards from the introspective point of view" (p. 331). Strong (1895) took issue with Marshall and distinguished between the sensation of pain and the feeling of unpleasure:

> The word pain signifies not only (1) the feeling we have when the skin is cut or burnt . . .; but also (2) the feeling of displeasure excited in us by this and other experiences. . . . That pain *is* displeasure . . . is what I am inclined to doubt.
>
> *(p. 330)*

He redefined pain: "Physical pain is . . . a sensation which calls forth displeasure" (p. 347). Strong (1896) admitted that this thesis is "a bold assumption" (p. 68). The neurological study of this skin sense produced pain that is not always displeasurable (McKeag, 1902; Strong, 1895). Strong's differentiation between the sensation of pain and the feeling of unpleasantness began an analysis of pain that orders discourses on pain to this day (see Osborn & Derbyshire, 2010) – an analysis based on the existence of something called "real pain."

To the extent that pain became constructed as a sensation, many pains in the vernacular sense were excluded from that category if their sensory cause could not be located. The traditional view, which spoke of sensory, emotional, aesthetic, and moral pains, viewed them all as pain. In the experimental discourse, non-real pain appeared. Along with real pain, "subjective pain" (McKeag, 1902, p. 61) became recognized, meaning pain allegedly originating in cortical centers rather than in the periphery. According to Luckey (1895), Goldscheider distinguished "real pain sensations" and "unreal, indirect, or pseudo-pains," the latter category including "pains occurring in sickness . . . most headaches, many stomach pains, etc." (p. 122). A third class of "psychic" pains exists, as found "in . . . neurasthenia, hysteria, hypochondria, etc." (p. 122). Psychic and physical (real) pains may combine, and real pain may produce psychic pain. Real pain "cannot properly be treated as the opposite of pleasure" (p. 123), but psychic pains can; like pleasures, they are feelings. This distinction between "real" and other pains became sedimented in psychology, medicine, public policy, and social representations.

Institutionalizing real pain

By 1900, the new psychology had defined pain as a sensation, although debate continued over its neurological correlates, some arguing that specific nerve endings produce pain, others arguing that a summation of sensory impulses produces pain. A majority, however, sided with the specific nerve version in the early twentieth century (Boring, 1942; Dallenbach, 1939). The sensation theory of pain, whatever its physiological explanation, was a better fit for the emerging natural scientific psychology rooted in physiology than was the quality theory.

The new view became institutionalized. In Baldwin's (1902) *Dictionary of Philosophy and Psychology*, pain arising from physical conditions was differentiated from "unpleasantness" (Vol. 2, p. 253). Titchener's *Textbook of Psychology* (1910) said that "the sensation obtained from the pain spots" (p. 152) on the skin

> are not necessarily painful. . . . The bright, itchy sensation and the sensation of prick occur as often as not in indifferent or pleasant complexes; it is only in the third stage, that of punctiform pain, that the sensation hurt.
>
> *(p. 155)*

Pain could be pleasant or unpleasant; an emotional overlay completes the experience of pain. Witmer (1894) cited a laboratory study that had produced a non-disagreeable pain: "The sensation of pain awakens no disagreeableness as long as we know that the harmful stimulus is only produced so as to call forth this feeling as an object of study" (Münsterberg, in Witmer, 1894, p. 222).

Objections remained. Titchener's (1908) dismissal of Marshall's theory provoked a reply from Marshall (1909b), who observed that Titchener himself noted that pain spots on the skin yield a variety of sensations, including itch, prick, sting, and then pain, so how can they be pain spots? Marshall also disputed the claim that pain as a sensation serves a useful biological warning function; what of "intestinal pains," "sciatica pains," and "tooth-nerve pains" (p. 9)? The latter alleged pain nerves only become activated when the damage is done, too late to warn of anything.

The advocates of experimental psychology readily adopted the sensation theory. Psychology textbooks literally inscribed the new theory into the skin of students (e.g., Singer, 1897). For example, in the work of Titchener (1901), pain spots located on a student's arm were mapped onto paper, and C. S. Myers (1911) used a needle and horsehair in classroom demonstrations. Mid-century textbooks (e.g., Jenkins, 1951) repeated that, in experimental settings, "mild stimulation of pain spots may not be painful at all" (p. 1178). Pain spots, when stimulated in certain ways, produce "painless pricks" or "a vague sense of stimulation" but not necessarily "true pain" (p. 1178).

Anatomizing real pain

Dallenbach (1939) observed that the sensation theory of pain had support, not only of physiological researchers but also of clinicians, especially Weir Mitchell and Henry Head. Head's famous self-experimentation, with the assistance of W.H.R. Rivers, deserves attention at this point, not only for the experiences described but also for the finer point made about the relations between psychology and physiology. In 1903, two surgeons made incisions in Head's left arm, and portions of the radial nerve and the cutaneous nerve were cut and then sutured together again:

> The following morning . . . the radial half of the back of the hand and dorsal surface of the thumb were found to be insensitive to stimulation with cotton wool, to pricking with a pin, and to all degrees of heat and cold.
>
> *(Rivers & Head, 1920, p. 226)*

Then followed a long series of experiments as the nerves regenerated. The experiments were psychophysical, as various stimuli (pin pricks, heat, cold, pressure, etc.) were brought into contact with the skin, and Head provided introspective reports of what he was feeling. These investigations revealed a protopathic sensibility, primitive and diffuse, which remained when the nerves in the study were severed, and an epicritical sensibility, more refined and specific, which gradually returned with the healing of the nerves. Rivers and Head claimed that the studies revealed the limits of a purely psychological analysis of sensation:

> Psychological analysis fails entirely to disclose the struggle of sensory impulses revealed by our experiment. Integration occurs as impulses pass

> from the periphery towards the higher centres; the change is a constant one from a complex to a simpler and more specific grouping. Sensation, the final end of the process, assumes forms simpler than any sensory impulses.
>
> *(p. 329)*

This meant that sensations are produced not as a direct line from the periphery to the center of the nervous system but as the impulses are integrated and inhibited as they pass from the periphery to the spinal cord. Physiological integration precedes the experience of sensibility.

On this account, the relationship between psychological and physiological investigation differed significantly from what Marshall proposed. For him, introspection was definitive, and the underlying corporeal processes had to conform to psychological investigation. Rivers and Head, while they used introspection to obtain their findings about sensibility, hypothesized that potential sensations never came into consciousness – they were not unconscious processes; they were purely physiological ones – except as they were transmitted to the brain, with much interaction occurring beforehand at both the peripheral level and in the spinal cord.

Such self-experimentation was repeated by others, and Head's conclusions regarding protopathic and epicritical pain were disputed. Wilfred Trotter and H. Morriston Davies (1909) reported similar self-experimentation. In discussing the means of observing the changes in the sensibility of the skin, Trotter and Davies pointed out that the methods used, such as the von Frey aesthesiometer, were not typical ways in which individuals perceive their skin and that this method could shape the resulting observations. In the end, Trotter and Davies disputed the protopathic/epicritical distinction for pain. Several years later, Edwin G. Boring (1916), trained in introspective psychology by Titchener, joined the debate; his self-study noted the following:

> Much has been made of the importance of the trained observer. It is doubtful, however, whether Head and Trotter and Davies, at least at the beginning of their experiments, were possessed of the introspective training which, in the psychological laboratory, would be considered adequate to their problem.
>
> *(p. 2)*

Even with the *qualê* theory no longer in play, the importance of introspection in terms of the self-observation of one's experience was critical in the study of cutaneous pain. Boring agreed with Trotter and Davies and rejected Head's hypothesis about the sequence of return of protopathic sensibility followed by that of epicritical sensibility. Reviewing the work of a half-century, Boring (1942) stated that "the fact seems to be that Head's theory has gradually dropped out of the textbooks while von Frey's has stayed" (p. 474). So at mid-century, the notion that specific nerves mediated cutaneous pain – the von Frey theory based upon Müller's doctrine – was the accepted version.

Sherrington's contributions

Charles S. Sherrington, the noted physiologist, physician, and philosopher, weighed in on pain in a chapter on cutaneous sensations (Sherrington, 1900). He drew on psychological and philosophical considerations as well as on physiological and medical considerations. He explicitly considered Marshall's thesis, objecting to the *qualê* theory on the grounds that the pain of a cut on a finger is not the same pain as that produced by musical discord. He distinguished pleasant and unpleasant feeling tones from physical pain, calling pain one form of the disagreeable. At the same time, he felt that the jury was still out on specific pain nerves. Sherrington decided: "This word [pain] will be here limited to phenomena of which everyday parlance speaks as bodily or 'physical' pain. 'Painful' is the affective colour of many psychical states" (pp. 968–969). Once the considerations were physiological and psychophysical, this limitation made sense. We see here most clearly the making of pain in the twentieth-century sense as pain connected with tissue damage.

Implications for the treatment of pain

The construction of pain that developed in psychology and medicine in the first half of the twentieth century was determined by the late nineteenth-century debates over pain. Pain was now thoroughly rooted in the anatomical image of the body, in its neurological details. Anesthesia and analgesics helped make that rootedness sensible. Pain was no longer tied to pleasure; pain was distinct from displeasure. Real pain had been constructed.

As a bridge between experimental psychology and medicine at the turn of the century, Witmer's (1897) contribution to the medical encyclopedia *Practice* can serve as an example. Witmer surveyed the neurology of pain, including arguments over specific nerve endings, and speculations about cortical and subcortical centers for pain. He saw the stakes as high, and he brought a fresh argument for the emphasis on pain paths in the nervous system:

> The notion that pain is a "purely subjective condition," a "feeling," "a state of mind without any physical basis in the body," may modify the attitude of a physician even in treating the simpler ailments of mankind. How much more may we expect the attitude of the neurological clinician towards pain to modify his views of the localization and causation of a disorder which may present pain disturbances as the most important symptoms! Thus we find Starr treating an "hysterical pain" by hypnotic suggestion, and maintaining it to be "subconscious, subjective, mental, without any physical basis," an opinion which has its roots in "rational psychology," finds modern representation in Janet's well-considered theories of psychic automatisms, and runs riot in Myers' notion of hysteria as a disease of the subconscious self.
>
> *(p. 903)*

For Witmer, what psychology can best do – and avoid the misconceptions that Dana drew from Marshall's work, a point Witmer reiterated (p. 904) – is to supply "physiology with a working hypothesis for the explanation of its own data, carefully refraining from the imposition of speculative data" (p. 904). The new psychology, as opposed to what Witmer called Marshall's "traditional psychology," sought neurological action wherever there was mental action. Without such evidence, a patient's complaints would not be taken seriously.

Witmer separated pain from unpleasant, subjective feelings. For Witmer, pain was a sensation, and the pleasant and the unpleasant were feelings based on motor reflexes of attraction and repulsion. He concluded that the specific organs for pain are probably in the spinal cord and cortical centers. Pain can thus be stimulated by "normal physiological processes, by spinal or cortical association, by irritation due to disease" (p. 941) and by other causes. Associations between pain and other stimuli, a type of learned pain, were possible, especially in cases of referred pain (pain felt in parts of the body distant from the source of the pain). In this construction of pain, the principal interpretative device is to look to the nervous system as imaged anatomically and in accord with the medical gaze.

We can conclude with Richard J. Behan's (1922) book *Pain*. Behan was a physician, and this book was directed at physicians. Behan's book may be said to have presented a consensus – medical common sense. Arney and Bergen (1983) cite Behan to illustrate how medicine from the late nineteenth to the mid-twentieth centuries conceptualized and treated disease with the medical gaze by anatomizing the disease: Behan's text looked at pain in relation to the various organ systems of the body, not in terms of patient narratives.

Behan (1922) referred to and dismissed Marshall's *qualê* view, and he helped sediment the distinction between real pain and subjective pain. Real pain is objective pain caused by injury or evident disease; subjective pain is mental pain. "Subjective pains," Behan wrote, "are those which have no physical cause for existence, but are the product of mental action arising from some changes of the coördinating centers of the sensorium" (p. 74). These pains occur in "emotional states, hysteria, habitual reactions, depressions of various types, compulsion neuroses, etc." (p. 74). They have "no organic basis for their presence, but may be the product of deranged mentality" (p. 74). An emotional pain entails sensations that are not really pain but rather "a feeling of unpleasantness" (p. 76). While he did warn against an overdiagnosis of hysteria, as real pain and real diseases could thereby be missed, he did distinguish hysterical pain from "real pain" (p. 79). Most significantly, Behan described "habit pains" – what today would be called chronic pain:

> This is the name given to that great class in which the pathways for pain have been so grooved from frequent repetition that on the least provocation the stimulus travels over them and gives rise to pain sensation. These frequently follow a trauma which has occurred some time previously. . . . Habit-pains frequently persist after operations of various kinds which have

> been undertaken because of the pain, and continue in spite of the fact that all the abnormalities have been corrected.
>
> *(p. 80)*

Habit pain, to stress the point, is not real pain, even though the nerves have been grooved and so readily respond to new stimuli. This is not real pain because it does not arise from observable damage to the objectified body. Now that pain is a sensation, some of what would have previously been understood to be pains were no longer pains. Behan stated that objective pain "always is the result of some demonstrable pathological change" (p. 82). Real pain existed in the Cartesian space of the anatomized corpse.

A Cartesian space of pain

The discovery of pain nerves "is one of the most important determinations happening within the epoch of Modern Psychology" (Nichols, 1896, p. 309) and a decisive break from "time-honored superstitions." For the 1893 World's Columbian Exposition in Chicago, Joseph Jastrow included a psychology laboratory in order to perform tests of sense and motion on visitors, including tests of "the typical forms of dermal sensation, pressure, roughness and smoothness, contact, pain" (in Sokal, 1973, p. 282). The sensation of pain was one of the fruits of a modern and scientific civilization.

A drawing from Descartes' 1644 treatise *Of Man* showing a nerve pathway from a man's foot to his brain has been used repeatedly to illustrate the sensation theory of pain. Melzack and Wall (1965), whose work did much to undermine this theory, pointed to the picture: "To call a receptor a 'pain receptor' . . . is a psychological assumption; it implies a direct connection from the receptor to a brain center where pain is felt" (p. 971). The illustration depicts a particular construction of pain. The Cartesian image implies a direct relationship between an interior space of the body and an external material world, the source of sensations. In fact, there are two types of interiors: that of the body and that of the soul which, in the Cartesian image, communicates with the brain. The inside and the outside of the body belong to a homogeneous space, the skin being a partition in objectified space. A direct communication occurs between the outside and the inside, although the qualities of the outside have to be transmitted in terms of the "specific nerve energies." Cartesian space is homogeneous, but it is compartmentalized into two regions: inside and outside the body.[1]

This Cartesian space of pain, which was in fact that of the first half of the twentieth century and not of the seventeenth century, was a divisible space. Since pain existed in that space as a signal, it could be interrupted: The foot could move, a researcher could section a nerve, a physician could inject a nerve block, the soul could distract its attention. Above all else, pain *signaled*: It represented danger in the external world or damage to the body. Each region of this divisible space had its professional caretakers. Physicians anatomized the body, and moralists anatomized the soul.

The biomedical model was constructed over the second half of the nineteenth century and the first half of the twentieth century. The medical gaze became progressively sharpened. Bonica (1990) wrote that "the widespread acceptance of the sensation theory led to the development and widespread use of regional analgesia and neurosurgical operations for the treatment of nonsurgical pain" (p. 11). What developed were ways that interfered with the signals from the periphery to the brain (see Bonica, 1953). Techniques included "nerve blocks" and the use of surgical anesthetics in the treatment of painful conditions. Between 1910 and 1920, the nerve block began to be used as an aid in the diagnosis, prognosis, and treatment of visceral pain and other diseases (Bonica, 1953, p. 172). Leriche, who did much to promote the idea of pain as a disease, used the sympathetic nerve block for relief of pain related to certain disorders. Between 1930 and 1950, nerve block clinics began to appear (Bonica, 1953, p. 180). In addition to these chemical "cuts" in Cartesian space, surgery for pain appeared at the same time, in the last quarter of the nineteenth century (Rey, 1993).

Inside the "pineal gland"

Biomedical treatments sought to block the pathways of pain in the space defined between the toe and the brain of the Cartesian image. It was understood, however, that not all pain would yield to such interventions. Left out of the picture was the place where pain actually occurred. For Descartes, that was the soul. No group aspiring to professional status in the nineteenth or twentieth centuries would actually call it by that name. In 1953, Bonica gave the contraindications for nerve blocks:

> Neurasthenic and psychoneurotic individuals are poor candidates for therapeutic blocks unless psychotherapy is employed in conjunction with the block. In patients with psychosomatic or psychogenic pain blocks should be avoided, because they are of no therapeutic value and occasionally will aggravate the condition.
>
> *(p. 179)*

The domain of functional disorders, of neurasthenia, of neurosis, of psychosomatics, produced pains that eluded the knife and the injection.

Critical reflections

The sensation theory of pain, and the treatments that it made possible and legitimate, ultimately rested upon the anatomical image of the body. Pain was translated into this image, into this symbolic form. As a result, the problems of psychogenic pain arose: the problem of the "two pains" and the growing problem of the invisibility of pain.

Real pain proved a questionable reality. As it permeated the broader society, the notion that some pains were imaginary and not real found uneasy affirmation. Swinburne (1907) wrote that suggestion can produce "imaginary pain. . . . The subjective mind . . . went along the line of the present environment, due to the emotional rather than the physical senses." Such pain suggested to patients in a dentist's office was thus not real because it arose from fear preceding any dental procedure. Phantom limb pain was also called "imaginary pain" because the arm, where the pain was felt, was not there (Hall, 1912). However, Hirschberg (1916) called "imaginary pains" the product of hallucinations (on analogy with visual hallucinations). Even though such pain is "not due to the usual realities of nature," such a pain is "an honest-to-goodness-cross-your-heart ache." What contradicted the sensation theory was often the testimony of individuals who, even if insane, as Hirschberg noted, still feel pain: "In your cosmos there is something to incite the sense of pain." The instability of the sensation theory contributed to its demise, as we shall see in the next chapter.

Ironic perhaps was the finding, noted by Luckey (1895), that stimulation of pain nerves produced pain only under certain conditions; other sensations resulted under other conditions. The irony was that the very method – introspection – that the sensation theory displaced was the very condition of possibility for knowing if these were indeed pain nerves. They were pain nerves because individuals experienced pain when they were stimulated in the right way. But then, if the experience did not include the stimulation of such nerves, the phenomenon was not real pain.

Marshall (1895b) complained that "too much emphasis is given to-day in some quarters to the physiological basis of psychology" (p. 60). Along these lines, Marshall noted that we regard pain but not pleasure as being problematic: "We set for ourselves these problems as to the existence of Pain, Error, Evil and Ugliness only because of a deep seated conviction that they display marked unrealness, and that Pleasure, Truth, Goodness and Beauty are more real" (1909b, pp. 399–400). Pain is thus a *privatio bonum* rather than a useful signal of tissue damage. And it is no accident, then, that Marshall, while not discounting a functional view of pain, had a more ample view, taking into account its uselessness – and thus sounding more contemporary.

Related to this expanded conception of pain is the relationship of the self and pain, which Marshall's work draws to our attention. He approvingly cites Herbert Spencer's definition that pain is "a feeling which we seek to get out of consciousness and to keep out" (Spencer, quoted in Marshall, 1920, p. 135). Consequently, the self "rejects and fails to assimilate what is painful" (Marshall, 1909b, p. 591). The telos of pain is unreality:

> Pain in connection with a given presentation involves a tendency to the failure of this presentation in attention, and this failure must tend to involve, in the moments to follow, the instability of the presentation which will give it unrealness.
>
> *(1909b, p. 397)*

Because of this tendency, pain is problematic. Pain should not be. Marshall did not claim that pain is unreal; he claimed that it *ought* not to be.

Marshall's psychology of pleasure and pain aimed at the clarification of concepts basic to the discipline, no matter how it is conceived – as a natural science, as a human science, as a social science, as a loosely configured set of studies – and the polemics of a century ago keep both the narrow question of pain and the broader question of the nature of psychology alive.

The construction of real pain ties into our larger theme as well. Pain became real pain when there was objective – meaning clearly visible to another – causes for it. When pain could be placed within a context of the anatomical body and objective conditions, then it was real. As Moscoso (2012) states, this entailed eliminating "subjective elements" (p. 96). The adjective *real*, displaced from objective conditions – and so constituting "real danger" – and onto pain itself, located some pain in the objective world. This move eclipsed meaning for the person in the process and "allowed for the elimination of subjective elements from the practice of medicine" (p. 86). Pain was spatialized in a depersonalized world.

Note

1 This section was drawn partially from Kugelmann (1997).

References

Arney, W. R., & Bergen, B. J. (1983). *Medicine and the management of living: Taming the last great beast.* Chicago, IL: University of Chicago Press.

Bain, A. (1887). On feeling as indifference. *Mind, 12*, 576–579.

Bain, A. (1892). Pleasure and pain. *Mind, New Series, 1*, 161–187.

Baldwin, J. M. (Ed.). (1902). *Dictionary of philosophy and psychology.* New York, NY: Macmillan.

Behan, R. J. (1922). *Pain: Its origin, conduction, perception and diagnostic significance.* New York, NY: Appleton.

Bonica, J. J. (1952). Management of intractable pain with analgesic blocks. *Journal of the American Medical Association, 150*, 1581–1586.

Bonica, J. J. (1953). *The management of pain.* Philadelphia, PA: Lea & Febiger.

Bonica, J. J. (1990). History of pain concepts and therapies. In J. J. Bonica (Ed.), *The management of pain* (2nd ed., Vol. 1, pp. 2–17). Philadelphia, PA: Lea & Febiger.

Boring, E. G. (1916). Cutaneous sensation after nerve division. *Quarterly Journal of Experimental Physiology, 10*, 1–95.

Boring, E. G. (1942). *Sensation and perception in the history of experimental psychology.* New York, NY: Appleton-Century.

Bradley, F. H. (1887). Association and thought. *Mind, 12*, 354–381.

Bradley, F. H. (1888). On pleasure, pain, desire and volition. *Mind, 13*, 1–36.

Calkins, M. W. (1916). *An introduction to psychology* (2nd ed.). New York, NY: Macmillan.

Cecil, H. (1910). *Liberty and authority.* London: Arnold.

Collins, J. (1894). Review of the book *Pain, Pleasure and Aesthetics* by Henry Rutgers Marshall. *Journal of Nervous and Mental Disease, 19*, 272–276.

Dallenbach, K. M. (1937). Herbert Nichols: 1852–1936. *American Journal of Psychology, 49*, 320–321.

Dallenbach, K. M. (1939). Pain: History and present status. *American Journal of Psychology, 52*, 331–347.

Danziger, K. (1980). The history of introspection reconsidered. *Journal of the History of the Behavioral Sciences, 16*, 241–262.

Danziger, K. (1990). *Constructing the subject: Historical origins of psychological research.* Cambridge, England: Cambridge University Press.

Danziger, K. (1996). The practice of psychological discourse. In C. F. Graumann & K. J. Gergen (Eds.), *Historical dimensions of psychological discourse* (pp. 17–35). Cambridge, England: Cambridge University Press.

Finger, S. (1994). *Origins of neuroscience: A history of explorations into brain function.* New York, NY: Oxford University Press.

Garvey, C. R. (1929). List of American psychology laboratories. *Psychological Bulletin, 26*, 652–660.

Griffing, H. (1896). On individual sensibility to pain. *Psychological Review, 3*, 412–415.

Griffing, H. (1897). Review of the book *Untersuchungen ueber die Sinnesfunctionen der menschlichen Haut. Erste Abhandlung; Druckempfindung und Schmerz. Psychological Review, 4*, 564–566.

Hacking, I. (1995). *Rewriting the soul: Multiple personality and the sciences of memory.* Princeton, NJ: Princeton University Press.

Hall, S. (1912, March 6). Development of Gadsden Purchase. *Weekly Journal-Miner*, p. 4. Retrieved from http://chroniclingamerica.loc.gov/

Hirschberg, L. K. (1916, November 7). Pain is felt close to trouble seat, not, as many believe, in brain. *Washington Times*, p. 8. Retrieved from http://chroniclingamerica.loc.gov/

James, W. (1892). A plea for psychology as a "natural science." *Philosophical Review, 1*, 146–153.

James, W. (1894, July 19). Marshall's pain and pleasure. *The Nation, 59*(1516), pp. 49–51.

Jenkins, W. L. (1951). Somesthesis. In S. S. Stevens (Ed.), *Handbook of experimental psychology* (pp. 1172–1190). New York, NY: Wiley.

Keele, K. D. (1957). *Anatomies of pain.* Springfield, IL: Thomas.

Kugelmann, R. (1997). The psychology and management of pain: Gate control as theory and symbol. *Theory & Psychology, 7*, 43–65.

Luckey, G.W.A. (1895). Some recent studies of pain. *American Journal of Psychology, 7*, 108–123.

Marshall, H. R. (1889). The classification of pleasure and pain. *Mind, 14*, 511–536.

Marshall, H. R. (1891a). The physical basis of pleasure and pain. I. *Mind, 16*, 327–354.

Marshall, H. R. (1891b). The physical basis of pleasure and pain. II. *Mind, 16*, 470–497.

Marshall, H. R. (1892). Pleasure-pain and sensation. *Philosophical Review, 1*, 625–648.

Marshall, H. R. (1894a). Are there special nerves for pain? *Journal of Nervous and Mental Diseases, 19*, 71–84.

Marshall, H. R. (1894b). *Pleasure, pain, and aesthetics.* New York, NY: Macmillan.

Marshall, H. R. (1895a). Physical pain. *Psychological Review, 2*, 594–598.

Marshall, H. R. (1895b). Pleasure, pain and emotion. *Psychological Review, 2*, 57–64.

Marshall, H. R. (1909a). Algedonics and sensationalism. *Journal of Philosophy, Psychology, and Scientific Methods, 6*, 5–13.

Marshall, H. R. (1909b). *Consciousness.* New York, NY: Macmillan.

Marshall, H. R. (1920). *Mind and conduct.* New York, NY: Scribner's.

McKeag, A. J. (Ed.). (1902). *The sensation of pain and the theory of specific nerve energies* (Vol. 2). Boston, MA: Ginn.

Melzack, R., & Wall, P. D. (1965). Pain mechanisms: A new theory. *Science, 150*, 971–979.

Mill, J. S. (1863). *Utilitarianism.* London, England: Parker, Son and Bourn.

Morris, D. (1991). *The culture of pain.* Berkeley: University of California Press.

Moscoso, J. (2012). *Pain: A cultural history* (S. Thomas & P. House, Trans.). New York, NY: Palgrave Macmillan.

Myers, C. S. (1911). *A text-book of experimental psychology with laboratory exercises.* New York, NY: Longmans, Green.

Nichols, H. (1892a). The origin of pleasure and pain. I. *Philosophical Review, 1,* 403–432.

Nichols, H. (1892b). The origins of pleasure and pain. II. *Philosophical Review, 1,* 518–534.

Nichols, H. (1896). Pain nerves. *Psychological Review, 3,* 309–316.

Norrsell, U., Finger, S., & Lajonchere, C. (1999). Cutaneous sensory spots and the 'law of specific nerve energies': History and development of ideas. *Brain Research Bulletin, 48,* 457–465.

Osborn, J., & Derbyshire, S.W.G. (2010). Pain sensations evoked by observing injury in others. *Pain, 148,* 268–274. http://dx.doi.org/10.1016/j.pain.2009.11.007

Rabinbach, A. (1990). *The human motor: Energy, fatigue, and the origins of modernity.* New York, NY: Basic Books.

Rey, R. (1993). *The history of pain* (L. E. Wallace, J. A. Cadden, & S. W. Cadden, Trans.). Cambridge, MA: Harvard University Press.

Rivers, W.H.R., & Head, H. (1920). A human experiment in nerve division. In H. Head (Ed.), *Studies in neurology* (Vol. 1, pp. 225–329). London, England: Hodder & Stoughton.

Santayana, G. (1894). Review of H. R. Marshall, *Pain, Pleasure, and Aesthetics. Psychological Review, 1,* 411–415.

Schiller, F. (1990). The history of algology, algotherapy, and the role of inhibition. *Pubbicazioni della Stazione Zoologica di Napoli, Section II: History and Philosophy of the Life Sciences, 12,* 27–50.

Sherrington, C. S. (1900). Cutaneous sensations. In E. A. Schäfer (Ed.), *Textbook of physiology* (Vol. 2, pp. 920–1001). Edinburgh, Scotland: Pentland.

Singer, E. A. (1897). Studies in sensation and judgment. *Psychological Review, 4,* 250–271.

Smith, R. (2013). *Between mind and nature: A history of psychology.* London, England: Reaktion Books.

Sokal, M. M. (1973). APA's first publication: Proceedings of the American Psychological Association, 1892–1893. *American Psychologist, 28,* 277–292. http://dx.doi.org/10.1037/h0038086

Stout, G. F. (1899). *A manual of psychology.* New York, NY: Hinds & Noble.

Strong, C. A. (1895). The psychology of pain. *Psychological Review, 2,* 329–347.

Strong, C. A. (1896). Physical pain and pain nerves. *Psychological Review, 3,* 64–68.

Swinburne, R. C. (1907, January 12). Suggestion as a medicine in dentistry. *The Daily East Oregonian,* p. 6. Retrieved from http://chroniclingamerica.loc.gov/

Syringo-myelia: Central glioma of the spinal cord, with spontaneous central hemorrhage. (1894). *Journal of Nervous and Mental Disease, 19,* 67–70.

Titchener, E. B. (1901). *Experimental psychology: A manual of laboratory practice* (Vol. I, Part II: Instructor's manual). New York, NY: Macmillan.

Titchener, E. B. (1908). *Lectures on the elementary psychology of feeling and attention.* New York, NY: Macmillan.

Titchener, E. B. (1910). *A textbook of psychology.* New York, NY: Macmillan.

Trotter, W., & Davies, M. (1909). Experimental studies in the innervation of the skin. *Journal of Physiology, 38,* 134–246.

Ward, J. (1887). Psychological principles III. *Mind, 12,* 45–67.

Witmer, L. (1894). The psychological analysis and physical basis of pleasure and pain. *Journal of Nervous and Mental Diseases, 19,* 209–228.

Witmer, L. (1897). Pain. In T. L. Stedman (Ed.), *Practice: An international encyclopedia of modern medical science, Vol. XI* (pp. 903–944). New York, NY: Wood.

Wolfe, H. K. (1895). The new psychology in undergraduate work. *Psychological Review, 2*, 382–387.

Wozniak, R. H. (1993). Theoretical roots of early behaviourism: Functionalism, the critique of introspection, and the nature and evolution of consciousness. In R. H. Wozniak (Ed.), *Theoretical roots of early behaviourism* (pp. ix–liii). London, England: Routledge/Thoemmes.

3

CONSTRUCTING PAIN NONDUALISTICALLY

Although the sensation theory defeated Marshall's, the old issues lingered, because even if pain nerves exist, pain is not only a sensation. Indeed, Marshall's *qualê* theory – but not his physiological speculations – continued to be invoked over the decades. The edges of Marshall's theory became softened, and no one proposed an algedonic *qualê*. What remained after the specifics were lost was a notion that pain had something to do with feeling and emotion. Referring to Marshall, Sherrington (1900) kept the debate alive, as did Dallenbach (1939), Beecher (1959), and Merskey and Spear (1967), who wrote that "the most obdurate resistance to the sensory theories came from H. R. Marshall and to some extent from C. A. Strong" (p. 8). Merskey and Spear referred to Marshall's view that either pain or pleasure must be part of any conscious experience. They affirmed that, with the sensation theory, the psychological character of pain was forgotten: "Pains became either 'real,' i.e. due to organic or functional afflictions of the nerves, or else imaginary" (p. 9). In the middle of the twentieth century, Merskey and Spear, along with Melzack, Wall, Fordyce, and others, reconstructed pain theoretically, arguing against a "Cartesian dualism" that had produced real and imaginary pain. Instead of constructing pain as a simple sensation, pain became a complex type of experience and a form of behavior. Did these efforts successfully eliminate dualism, whatever that might mean?

Cartesian dualism and pain

A so-called Cartesian dualism haunts psychological conceptions of pain, and it frames everyday discourse of pain. Scientific theories, especially before the middle of the century, considered pain "an unintentional sensation, a physiological process 'happening' in the body without any subject" (Honkasalo, 2000, p. 197). In this formulation, pain is a warning signal caused by stimulation of certain sensory nerves, indicating tissue damage. Such pain is "real pain." Subjectivity enters as emotional and cognitive reactions to the pain sensation. People reporting pain in the absence of tissue damage do not have real pain – they have psychogenic pain. Psychogenic pain is emotional displeasure, not really pain, for which physical damage provides legitimizing evidence.

This Cartesian dualism exists in social representations as well. Jean E. Jackson (1994) found it among patients in a pain clinic: "Most of us tend to think of pain as something physical: since we experience pain in the body, in so far as we see our bodies as physical objects, so will we see pain as physical" (p. 207). Gillian Bendelow and Simon Williams (1995) contended that pain "has been 'medicalized,' resulting in the inevitable Cartesian split between body and mind" (p. 84). Gillies and her colleagues (2004) found Cartesianism in their own ways of experiencing pain, and they observed that sometimes dualism was helpful in dealing with pain by providing a distance between self and pain. Such a finding should add a note of caution to calls to overcome Cartesianism.

This dualism is not only a theoretical issue; it is political as well. Wailoo (2014) describes the debates over disability assistance in the post–World War II era, when there was significant disagreement over the nature of pain and whether more harm was done in providing assistance to veterans or in denying them benefits – since some believed that assistance could make them dependent on government benefits. In part, the debates turned on the nature of real pain. One psychiatrist in 1957 worried about "liberalized disability relief" (p. 49) and claimed that people with psychogenic pain "were simply maladjusted malingerers" (p. 49). For Wailoo, "pain in all its confusing duplicity had arrived – a mysterious, worrisome presence in postwar society" (p. 53). With psychoanalytic ideas dominating psychiatry at that time, psychogenic pain became a political football: "Psychologizing of the pain complaint became common fare as critics linked liberal medicine to an insidious social and political threat" (p. 55). With this background in mind, we turn to challenges to real pain in the 1960s.

Despite widespread acceptance of "real pain," there were anomalies that it could not explain, such as wounds unaccompanied by pain and pain persisting after the tissue damage had healed. Such anomalies led to parallel attempts in the middle of the twentieth century to overcome Cartesian dualism in the conception of pain. This chapter considers three such efforts in the mid-twentieth century: (1) the gate control theory of pain, which sought to integrate sensory and psychological factors in a neuropsychological conception of pain; (2) a psychosomatic approach that argued that people describe both physical and psychogenic pains in identical terms; and (3) a behavioral approach to the treatment of pain, which sought to bypass the real–imaginary dichotomy by focusing on pain behavior as a learned response to environmental reinforcement.

Gate control: a technological construction of pain[1]

The sensation theory has two variations: the specificity theory, which proposed pain nerves, and the pattern theory, which asserted that intensity of stimulation and patterns of peripheral nerve action signaled pain. The specificity theory, Ronald Melzack and Patrick Wall (1965) stated and Wall (1996) reiterated, was a Cartesian "scheme of sensation created by pulling on a rope, which rang the pain bell" (p. 18). Whatever this sensation theory owes to Descartes, it was not, as we have seen, the way to envision pain until around the year 1900. In this spatialized world of pain, pain paths could be visualized, and mechanical and chemical ways were found to block messages to the brain. However, surgical and other disruptions of pain pathways were not always successful. William K. Livingston, a surgeon at the University of Oregon Medical School, noted the limitations of the specificity theory in stating: "I have been increasingly impressed with the *dynamic* characteristics of pain, its urgency and its remarkable ability to find a new route when the customary channels have been blocked" (1943/1976, p. 26; italics in the original). In this regard, pain is like memory. Memory can be "temporarily abolished by a wide variety of lesions but persistently returns in all but devastating lesions" (p. 18). Livingston found the same re-emergence of pain after its pathways had been severed. Wall (1996) lamented the dangers posed by the specificity theory in caustic terms:

> The one remaining, and apparently immortal and indestructible, virtue of specificity theory is its utter simplicity. It has failed to generate any explanation for clinical pains. It has failed to generate any usable therapy and, worse, has encouraged ineffective, often counterproductive, surgical attempts to destroy the cells or their axons.
>
> *(p. 17)*

This critique of Cartesianism in the theory of pain had implications for the distinction between physical and psychogenic pain.

Melzack studied psychology with Donald Hebb, a theorist interested in the brain's role in learning. From Hebb, Melzack learned a conception of psychology different from the stimulus–response psychology of the likes of Skinner, dismissed as a "model of a telephone switchboard system" (Oral History Interview, 1993, p. 11), using the same imagery which, when applied to pain, is the Cartesian sensation theory. For Hebb (1949), the brain mediated between stimulus and response, although Hebb reached no conclusions about the nature of neural activity underlying pain. When Melzack reconsidered his early paper on dogs raised in isolation that did not seem to sense pain (Melzack & Scott, 1957), Melzack applied this Hebbian approach:

> I knew that they could feel pain, because in their home cages, they would respond to electric shock, but when they came out, somehow they would ignore it. And I came to the realization that the brain somehow had to receive information about what was going on in the outside world, but that was not the basis of a perception. The brain received this information, it evaluated that information, and then it would send messages down to some gating area, as I would call it now, where it would let the stuff in or keep it out.
>
> *(Oral History Interview, p. 12)*

After studies with Hebb, Melzack trained in physiology with Livingston. Later, at MIT, Melzack met Wall, a physiologist with an extensive background in electrophysiology, where work in physiology intersected engineering and computer science. Wall's interests included studying inhibitory mechanisms in the spinal cord. Wall recounted an incident that illustrated what he was finding in his investigations:

> One of my jobs was mowing vast acres of lawn with a hand-pushed motor mower with a hellish vibration. I began to realize that after enough vibration, my hands were really remarkably numb, and I thought well let's try that on a cat. So Cronly-Dillon and I published on the fact that vibration outside the receptive field of a cell would inhibit it. That was the first trigger for the gate control.
>
> *(An interview, 2015, p. 12)*

In the symbolic order of the time, where physiological and psychological discourses mixed with those of computers and electrical engineering (whose devices were significant in physiological research), Wall and Melzack proposed that a "gate" regulated the transmission of peripheral impulses signaling pain in the spinal cord. Wall explained the image of the gate:

> We were always using triode valves which had a gate. That was my meaning of the word gate. We'd been struggling with gate currents and used a gate control all the time for varying amplification. In that diagram [in Melzack & Wall, 1965] . . . I'd introduced the smallest number of possible components, and some pure guesswork like the fact that the proposal that the substantia gelatinosa was the origin of the inhibitory control.
>
> *(p. 12)*

The idea of inhibitory control led to the construction of a transcutaneous electrical nerve stimulation (TENS) device (Wall & Sweet, 1967), which controlled pain by inhibiting pain signals in the spinal cord. Such success helped convince many of the gate control theory. Indeed, the 1965 paper became "the most influential article in the field of pain" (Liebeskind, in *Oral History Interview*, 1993, p. 26).

The gate control theory significantly modified the sensation theory. When peripheral stimulation from pain nerves entered the spinal cord (where the "gate" was located), it combined with other peripheral stimulation and with inputs from the brain. In this way, memories, motivations, emotions, and cognitions could facilitate or inhibit the transmission of signals to the brain that resulted in the feeling (or not) of pain. The theoretical differences between physical and psychogenic pain, then, had to do with which input – peripheral or central – dominated in the resulting pain.

The gate control theory was inaccurate physiologically, and Merskey (1994) saw its significance primarily in symbolic terms, a point seconded by Wailoo

(2014), who indicated that the theory rested "on almost no experimental foundations" (p. 85). However, as Wall (1996) claimed, the theory "was not a bad guess for its time" (p. 16), pointing out that its idea has been generative of subsequent research. Indeed, "it had encouraged new pain interventions" (Wailoo, p. 85), including TENS. The schematic diagram that illustrated this new construction of pain depicted the contributions of the environment, sensory nerves, the central nervous system, personality, thoughts, memories, and expectations in the production of pain.

The gate control diagram (see Melzack, 1974, p. 276) exemplifies how this allegedly post-Cartesian world would map neurological, psychological, and social inputs on the same plane. Like the "biopsychosocial model" (Engel, 1977), with its chimera of holism resting on a biomedical foundation (Stam, 2015), the gate control model did not specify what "central control processes" and "motivational–affective processing" meant. The reader understands that these things mean both neurological activities – the activation of circuits in the brain and spinal cord – and psychosocial activities. The flowchart put the psychological and somatic components that existed in different regions of Cartesian space together in a process. Pain "does not consist of a single ring of the appropriate central bell, but is an ongoing process" (Melzack & Wall, 1965, p. 976). The gate control theory depicts chronological time, not Cartesian space, with its mental and physical regions. The new theory provided a kind of narrative, with differences between inside and outside, self and other, mind and body, integrated into circuits. The gate control theory sought to eliminate Cartesian dualism with circuits connecting the mental and the physical.

In other words, the gate control theory provided a new metaphor for pain. The metaphor asserts that pain is a process. Perl and Kruger (1996) noted that the gate control theory "was provocative in combining the terminology of digital electronics and the concept of presynaptic inhibition" (p. 190). The force of the metaphor is to make pain into a technical event. In accentuating process as technique, it invites a response that is equally technique oriented. Indeed, Wall (1996) confessed that

> I have grown steadily more allergic . . . to the facile borrowing of technological terms to submerge a combined ignorance of technology and biology. (In fact, I regret borrowing the word "gate" from triodes and transistors because it was interpreted as a switch).
>
> *(p. 19)*

Melzack also noted how the setting at MIT played a role in defining the theory – that is, a technological lifeworld provided a symbolic form for the new conception of pain:

> And if we were not at MIT, I'm not sure we would have used the "gate," the word, but we used a lot of engineering type terms in there, trying to keep it as simple as possible, so it really evolved. And "gating," the engineers were

> talking about "gating" all over the place, all those computer guys were talking about it, and computers were big anyway.
>
> *(Oral History Interview, p. 24)*

Whatever its limitations, the gate control theory reflected the emerging "high-tech" world of the mid-twentieth century, and it has proven to have staying power. It is still widely cited in textbooks as the model of pain, and some physicians refer to it as unquestionably true.

However, the specificity theory is not dead, with researchers such as Edward R. Perl contributing to its nuanced revival. Basbaum (2011), while not failing to mention that "the poster boy/dartboard for the specificity camp, of course, is Descartes' little boy whose 'pain pathway' runs from his foot to a pain center in his brain," cited research supporting the existence of "behaviorally relevant specificity, *at least at the level of the primary afferent*" (italics in the original). This specificity does not negate pain circuitry; it only further complicates it. Indeed, unlike Descartes' "pain pathway," pain is no bell ring:

> This contemporary perspective on the question of specificity versus patterning relates more to the processing of nociceptive messages, and much less so to the sensory experience/perception of pain. The latter is clearly influenced and in some cases dominated by emotional and cognitive factors.
>
> *(Basbaum, 2011)*

The experience of pain will be the result of these various processes.

An operational construction of pain

In the mid-1960s, around the same time that Melzack and Wall constructed the gate control theory, two British psychiatrists, Harold Merskey and Graham Spear, proposed an operational definition of pain based on studies of pain in psychiatric patients. The definition came from Merskey's (1964) doctoral dissertation: Pain is "an unpleasant experience which we primarily associate with tissue damage or describe in terms of tissue damage or both" (Merskey & Spear, 1967, p. 21). This definition became the basis of the International Association for the Study of Pain (IASP) definition of pain, to which was added a phrase giving a nod to the sensation theory: "an unpleasant *sensory and emotional* experience" (Merskey et al., 1979, p. 250; emphasis added). While Merskey and Spear (1967) briefly discussed the gate control theory, the definition that Merskey proposed preceded it and was, he stated, not tied to any theory of the causes of pain. His initial aim was to legitimize psychogenic pain as real pain.

Body image and psychogenic pain

Both Merskey and Spear worked under Erwin Stengel, a psychoanalyst, who in turn had studied under Paul Schilder and Sigmund Freud (Merskey, 2000) in

Vienna. Schilder had developed a concept of "body image" in psychoanalytical terms and had addressed the problem of pain (Szasz, 1957/1975, p. 78). Stengel (1965) recalled that after moving to Sheffield in 1957, he

> hoped that one or other of my younger colleagues would take an interest in problems of pain in psychiatric illness. I was very glad when Graham Spear and Harold Merskey working in my department embarked on research projects in this field.
>
> *(p. 798)*

Confining his remarks to "physical pain" only – dismissing "so-called mental pain, a vague concept referring to distress not related to the body" (p. 793) – Stengel asserted that "psychiatrists . . . have attempted, not very successfully, to distinguish clinically between organic and psychogenic pain" (p. 796). Psychogenic pain exists, in part, because "every sensation gets its sense and meaning only in connection with the whole body" (p. 797). Following Schilder,[2] for Stengel, regardless of its cause, psychogenic pain is physical pain, not mental pain. In his argument, he cited Merskey's definition of pain "as an unpleasant experience" (p. 798). The editor of the *British Journal of Psychiatry*, the psychiatrist Eliot Slater, questioned this use, asserting that pain was a sensation produced by the stimulation of pain nerves (Slater, 1966). For Slater, Merskey's definition produced confusion, because a great variety of unpleasant feelings might be called pain. In reply, both Stengel (1966) and Merskey (1966) urged that the language of psychology not be confused with that of physiology, with Stengel writing: "Pain due to psychological causes has the same significance for the patient as pain due to physical disturbance, and therefore the former has to resemble the latter subjectively" (p. 330). Different causes of pain do not lead to different experiences of pain. They found support in the work of Thomas Szasz: "Szasz has been a formidable critic of confused thinking about pain" (Merskey & Spear, 1967, pp. 17–18), especially the concept that pain has two components: the sensation and the emotional reaction to the sensation. Claiming to be able to separate out the sensation and the reaction can amount to situations in which "the patient's experience is, in fact, denied" (p. 18). They also found helpful Szasz's call to keep the languages of physiology and psychology distinct, even though the two are addressing the same phenomena (p. 24).

Szasz on pain and body image

Thomas Szasz was a psychoanalyst best known for his critiques of the psychiatric establishment and concepts of mental illness. In *Pain and Pleasure* (1957/1975), he argued that pain "is often a bodily feeling, but sometimes it is not" (p. 4). Pain could be a "sensation, perception, affect, signal, or 'object'" (p. 12). He held that pain concerns the relationship of the ego to the body, just as anxiety – from which pain is, early in development, undifferentiated – concerns the relationship of the ego with others. Therefore, pain is primarily an affect (p. 59). The "body" that the ego fears for in pain is the body image along the lines that Schilder (1950) described. The implication? "When we consider pain in terms of the relationship of the body to the ego, the distinction between 'organic' and 'psychogenic' automatically disappears" (p. 70). Why?

> From the point of view of the experiencing ego, all pain refers to the body. This highlights the fact that the terms "organic" and "psychogenic" do not, strictly speaking, refer to the pain experience at all but describe the judgment of the observer about the source or location of the pain.
>
> *(pp. 70–71)*

The way people perceive their bodies need not correspond to the anatomical image of the body. Instead, the perceived body corresponds to the body image or, in phenomenological terms, the lived body. Guided by Szasz, one may ask of a complaint of pain, which body, which body image, has been wounded? Sometimes, perhaps much of the time, it is a body image convertible into the anatomical image (see Szasz, 1957/1975, p. 73).

The body is not simply an object for oneself; it is also an object for others, so that bodily events are social events. Szasz (1957/1975) indicated the interpersonal meanings of pain and its expression: "It is a fundamental method of asking for help" (p. 86). In redefining pain as signifying a danger to the lived body (and not simply its anatomical image), Szasz moved away from the sensation theory. Nevertheless, he stated that bodily danger "refers to anatomical and physiological matters and will be designated accordingly as the *medical meaning* of pain" (p. 88; italics in the original). Pain as a call for help "refers to human relations and may be called the *communicative meaning* of pain" (p. 88; italics in the original). When physicians hear the communicative meaning as the medical meaning, they use medical treatment for an essentially nonmedical condition. Szasz's analysis indicated the extent to which the anatomical image underlies medical perception.

Engel and psychogenic pain

George Engel played a key role in the Merskey and Spear reformulation. Stengel (1965) noted the similarity between Engel and Merskey, observing that "Engel has furnished the only consistent theory of psychogenic pain" (p. 801). Engel (1959) argued against the received view that pain was primarily a sensation with affective overlays. His starting point was the observation that "what is experienced and reported as pain is a psychological phenomenon" (p. 916). On this basis, one cannot argue that the only real pain is that provoked by the stimulation of nociceptors. The notion of psychogenic pain is an improvement on assertions that a patient's pain is imaginary (p. 899). Engel pointed out that other sensory experiences occur without peripheral stimulation, as in sensory deprivation experiments. So with pain; it may occur as a result of peripheral activity, but it need not. Turning then to characteristics of pain, Engel observed that pain always has an affective aspect: "It is never neutral" (p. 901). The main focus of the Engel article was on the psychosocial characteristics of pain: In addition to being a biological warning signal, pain plays important roles in personal life. Its expression can lead to comfort and attention and relief; it can be administered as punishment; it is connected to "aggression and power" (p. 901) in the giving and receiving of it. Pain can develop when we lose or fear the loss of loved ones, and pain can satisfy the guilt over real or fantasized aggression toward loved ones. Finally, there are "pain-prone patients," people who develop a propensity for pain because it can "yield pleasure . . . in a relative sense, that is, in place of something even more distressing" (p. 902). Engel elaborated ways in which pain can play out in the psychic economy and the ways in which pain can wreak havoc in medical settings.

Psychosomatics: beyond the sensation theory

Early articles of Merskey, Spear, and others were published in the *Journal of Psychosomatic Research*, founded in 1956, with Denis Leigh as editor-in-chief. Leigh had a strong commitment to psychosomatic research, as the editorial for Volume 1 indicated:

> Psychosomatic medicine has as its objective the understanding of man, neither as an exclusively physical nor as an exclusively psychic being, but as an integrated totality. The term psychosomatic medicine is not altogether satisfactory, as it connotes a duality of body and mind rather than a body-mind unity. As yet, no satisfactory alternative term has been generally accepted to denote the modern conception of the field of psychosomatic medicine as comprising both body-mind unity and the organism-environment continuum.
>
> *("Editorial," 1967, p. 1)*

In this journal, Merskey and colleagues published a series of research papers that explored correlations between various psychopathologies and persistent pain. For the majority of the patients studied, the pain seemed to be psychogenic; nevertheless, the patients' descriptions of their pain resembled what nonpsychiatric patients say of their pain. Devine and Merskey (1965) found overall similarities in the descriptions of psychiatric and medical pain, with pain's symbolic and communicative value playing a role, and found that "such considerations will apply to the terms used to describe pain and that this remains true whether it is 'psychogenic' or 'organic' " (p. 315). Patient descriptions were more similar than otherwise:

> There was no difference in the types of description given by the patients whose pain was "organic" and by those whose pain was "psychogenic." . . . The persistence of the pain and its significance to the individual are likely to affect the description of it perhaps as much as or more than other causes.
>
> *(p. 316)*

This attention to what patients say – what Merskey (1965) called "the phenomenological characteristics of pain" (p. 291) – represented an important point of departure for the analysis of pain.

Merskey and Spear (1967) argued that while sensory and affective aspects can be distinguished abstractly, they doubted that this was possible in practice. Peripheral stimulation and a motor response to it are physiological components, but one cannot make the leap to saying that pain has two components: a sensory one and a reactive (emotional) one. The belief that peripheral stimulation is essential for pain is not true and, if believed, leads to negating many patients' experiences. Nevertheless, Merskey and Spear defended the use of the term *psychogenic pain* for practical reasons. Whereas organic pain following an injury appears self-evident to doctor and patient alike, pain without such an explanation still needs a name indicating its potential causes. The term *psychogenic pain* carries the risk of a belief that "a subjective difference can be established between the two types of pain" (p. 19). Patients describe what is called *psychogenic pain* "in terms of noxious stimuli or tissue damage" (p. 20). Merskey and Spear concluded that

> in view of the evidence that "organic" and "psychogenic" pains are frequently described in the same terms . . . and that the unpleasant characteristics of pain may be partly delimited from other unpleasant experiences, it is possible to give this operational definition of pain: "*An unpleasant experience which we primarily associate with tissue damage or describe in terms of tissue damage or both.*"
>
> *(p. 21; italics in the original)*

The purpose of calling this an operational definition is to "avoid the confusion which is frequently evident in the medical literature as to what constitutes pain" (p. 22). They stated that they were also seeking a philosophical position on pain – namely, a monistic one, following Szasz (1957/1975). Allowing for the validity of both physiological and psychological approaches to pain, they supported Szasz's view that using both together leads to a confusion of words and things. The terms *psychological* and *physiological* do not refer to distinct things but to distinct ways of describing the same thing.

Operationalizing: struggling with dualism

Merskey's definition sought to avoid the confusions created by dualist thinking, but it did make a concession to dualism. By including the phrase "describe in terms of tissue damage," Merskey and Spear acknowledged that when people want to be taken seriously about their pain, they refer to the body in a way that a physician would recognize. A person may say, *I have a headache* or *My back hurts.* The medical context signifies these statements in terms of the anatomical image of the body. This translation is problematic if the meaning of the pain in the person's life is not only about a physical injury. Merskey and Spear (1967) wrestled with the problem this creates: "We do not wish to suggest that pain is a phenomenon which is independent of bodily integrity, but we consider that this somatic bias has led to confusion and incompleteness in thinking and theorizing about pain" (p. 169). This somatic bias results from dualist thinking, particularly from its reduction of all pain to acute sensory pain. Merskey and Spear's way of handling this bias involved three decisions. First, they assumed mind–body identity – namely, that mental accounts and physiological accounts point to the same reality. Second, they pointed to two distinct discourses, one based on "data obtained from observation of the system from without (public data)" and the other based on "data which originate from within the system (private data) and are made public by a process of translation, normally, in this context, by the person who is the system under observation" (p. 170). This "translation" is typically into the language of biomedicine, which is the language common to the person and the observer. (If the observer were a practitioner of traditional Chinese medicine, then the translation might be very different.) Third, they stressed the importance of choice of discourse in a particular situation. Using psychological discourse will mean using "concepts of feelings and meanings rather than concepts of stimuli and physiological changes" (p. 170). The two discourses are "alternative descriptions and explanations of the same phenomenon" (p. 170). In the end, they affirmed Szasz's psychological theory that whatever the initial cause of pain, it can take on communicative and symbolic meanings and be maintained because those meanings matter to the person.

This way of recognizing dualism and trying to avoid it Merskey called *operationalizing*. Merskey (1994) later said that he found support for this in Stengel's work for the World Health Organization (WHO) in the 1950s. The WHO had had Stengel study why many countries failed to adopt the International Classification of Diseases (ICD-6) of 1948: "Stengel suggested that the solution was to develop a classification that simply provided operational definitions of mental disorders without reference to etiology" (Keeley, Morton, & Blashfeld, 2015, pp. 45–46). Stengel (1959) drew on the philosophical work of Carl G. Hempel (1965) to argue for a classificatory system of mental disorders for diagnostic purposes without attempting to organize it along theoretical lines. Surveying a veritable Tower of Babel of classificatory systems around the globe, Stengel wrote:

> There is much to be said in favour of operational definitions in psychiatry. . . . Schizophrenia, then, as an operational definition, would not be an illness, or a specific reaction type, but an agreed operational definition for certain types of abnormal behavior. It should be less difficult to agree about an operational definition than about a hypothetical illness. . . . The question . . . is not what schizophrenia or psychopathy is, but what interpretation should be placed on these concepts for the purpose of diagnosis and classification, i.e., for the purpose of communication.
>
> *(p. 612)*

Since pain was also subject to theoretical disputes, and since the dichotomy of organic and psychogenic pains persisted, having an operational definition of pain that relied on what a patient said or did (the phrasing "describe in terms of tissue damage" not implying that the patient had to be the one doing the describing [Anand & Craig, 1996]) enabled communication and assumed the credibility of the complaint. Hempel's essay on taxonomy, presented at the same conference where Stengel spoke, extended the meaning of operationalizing to include the kind of definition that Merskey provided:

> If the insistence on an *operational* specification of meaning for scientific terms is not to be unduly restrictive, the idea of operation has to be taken in a very liberal sense which does not require manipulation of the objects under consideration: the mere observation of an object, for example, must be allowed to count as an operation.
>
> *(Hempel, 1965, p. 143; italics in the original)*

In the case of pain, what is observed is a person saying that he or she is in pain – typically, one would assume, with corresponding movements and gestures, with the possibility (Merskey, 1994) that occasionally one will be deceived.

Constructing pain as behavior

If pain was to be operationalized, constructing pain as behavior seems to be a reasonable development. In the mid-1960s, a psychologist, Wilbur Fordyce, working with the anesthesiologist John J. Bonica at the University of Washington, introduced behavioral techniques for the treatment of pain. Adopting an innovation of Jack Michael's (Ayllon & Michael, 1959), which taught operant conditioning methods to psychiatric nurses working in a mental hospital to control patient behavior, "Fordyce made an effort to influence expressions of pain in a hospitalized patient by structuring attention or social feedback" (Fordyce, 1987, p. 313). This was the beginning of Fordyce's approach to pain as behavior, which has been widely applied in pain treatment programs, with more than a thousand programs in the United States alone by 1987 (p. 313).

Fordyce's conceptualization of pain resembled the psychosomatic approach that the behavioral approach displaced. Like Szasz, Engel, Merskey, and Spear, Fordyce argued that chronic pain was not always the symptom of an underlying organic pathology and that, even if it were, other factors were involved in maintaining it. Echoing Szasz and Engel, Fordyce (1988) observed that "pain behaviors are interesting social communications, the meanings of which remain to be discovered in the individual case" (p. 282). To conceptualize pain in behavioral terms meant to identify what a person does and says that indicates being in pain: "He may verbalize complaints, moan audibly, grimace, recline to await the termination of pain, assume a special posture to minimize the pain, seek distraction, or, perhaps, request the help of others, as in asking for pain relieving medication" (Fordyce, Fowler, Lehmann, & DeLateur, 1968, p. 179). These "signals," combined with the behavior that follows them, are "pain behaviors." Considering pain in this behavioral model rather than in the "medical model" produced new possibilities for the treatment of some chronic pain. This approach did not presume to deal with every aspect of pain: "Pain behavior, though not necessarily the peripheral signal which originally led to the pain behavior, is subject to the same set of laws and systems for modification as other kinds of behavior" (p. 180). The goals of treatment were fewer pain behaviors and increased productive activity. In particular, one goal was a reduction in the use of painkillers, and a second goal was more activity such as walking or participating in occupational therapy.

Fordyce did not assume that pain initially showed up because of reinforcement; however, the behavior that developed subsequently to the onset of pain was subject to learning. Significantly, as with the psychosomatic approach, the behavioral approach sought to avoid the implication that some pains were genuine and others were not:

> The issue of whether the pain a patient reports is "real" or otherwise is simply not relevant. In this context "real" means approximately that some neurophysiological defect or pathology can be demonstrated. . . . Characteristically, from the medical model, the alternative to an explanation of reported pain as being "real" is to attribute pain to so-called mental or psychical processes. Examples are represented by labels such as "hysterical," "suggestion," "imaginary," "hypochondriacal," or "secondary gain." . . . In contrast, the approach described in this paper focuses on modifying the pain behavior itself, however much or little "real" its origins were.
>
> *(Fordyce et al., 1968, p. 189)*

This behavioral approach was thus another way to address the limitations of the sensation theory. Like Merskey, Fordyce did not deal with the presumed causes of pain. The two approaches also did not deny the wide applicability of a medical model approach to the treatment of pain; they asserted, however, that medical treatment could be counterproductive. Finally, the two held, as did the gate control theory, that pain was not always a signal of danger or tissue damage and that it had interpersonal or social meanings. In other words, pain is an activity, something people do or make, and its significance, its exacerbation, and its relief come in many forms.

Fordyce's notion of pain does owe something to the sensation theory, even as it undermines it. In differentiating pain and suffering, Fordyce (1988) aligned pain with nociception (the perception of harmful stimuli), even if pain can happen without nociception and vice versa. He saw suffering as "an affective or emotional response in the central nervous system,[3] triggered by nociception *or* other aversive events, such as loss of a loved one, fear, or threat" (p. 278; italics in the original). Pain, whether or not it is triggered by nociception, is a "signal," and suffering, along with pain behavior, is a "response" (p. 278). This distinction returns to the two-component theory of pain – sensation and emotion – and Fordyce assumed that the two could be not only differentiated but also treated separately:

> The so-called pain experience is often a misidentification by the patient. He is getting a signal; he thinks it is a pain signal from the periphery when indeed it is something else. When that is the case, by using behavioral approaches, you can help him . . . take medication down, the activity level up, and the pain experience goes away.
>
> *("Floor Discussion," 1974, p. 592)*

The behavioral approach teaches that such an individual is not experiencing pain; it is something else, perhaps anxiety. This differentiation of sensation and response owed much to a stimulus–response view of behavior, and it was out of step with the more interactive view, as expressed by Wall (1996):

> It is no longer permissible to view perception as a self-contained process simply fed by a reliable apparatus. Cognitive expectations influence the operation of the sensory apparatus, thereby destroying the classically assumed isolation of a primary sensory mechanism, which is followed by a second isolated process, which is the operation of the mind.
>
> *(p. 15)*

The behavioral approach reverted to an empiricist theory of mind, in which sensation was a passive reception of stimuli.

A 1980s exchange debated the relative merits of an operant approach. While there was agreement that clinicians should not remain "fixed in the acute pain organic medical model" (Steger, 1981), Steger – a colleague of Fordyce at the University of Washington Medical School – asserted that Merskey underestimated learning factors in the production of some chronic pain, emphasizing personality factors instead. In reply, Merskey (1982) stated that while he did not reject Fordyce's learning theory approach, "[he] consider[ed] the strict operant approach, as distinct from the general supportive and management approaches of any psychiatrist or psychologist, to have little additional contribution to offer to the majority of pain patients." Moreover, "the strict operant approach neglects the experience of patients." Compared to what he thought was an "extreme view" of pain management, Merskey instead endorsed the position taken by Sternbach (1981, p. 162) that, while "pain reactions are modifiable," there are a variety of ways in which pain behavior is learned, leading to a variety of treatments – not only the operant one – including "social modelling." In addition, cognitive approaches, hypnosis, and psychodynamic therapy are treatment options. Fordyce (1983) replied to the charge that his approach neglected experience: If pain is what a patient reports, then behavioral techniques seek to influence those reports. Moreover, Fordyce continued: "If one perceives 'pain' as a class of events that can be inferred or measured only by what the person does (including what he or she says), a quite different set of conclusions follows." Merskey (1983, p. 731) then accused Fordyce of "trying somehow to revise the plain meaning used by most people, which is included in the IASP definition." The behaviorist redefinition of pain would restrict the meaning of pain statements to the way in which such statements act in the situation. For Merskey, however, that restriction of meaning occludes other types of signification.

The economics of pain behavior

To clarify this dispute between Merskey and Fordyce over the definition of pain, we turn to remarks Merskey (1994) made to John Liebeskind. According to Merskey, insurance companies promote behavioral approaches as a way of reducing costs by having people return to work. In itself, this is a desirable outcome. However:

> I think that there is a . . . tendency to believe that pain can be explained in behavioral terms. And the reason why that problem exists is because of the insurance system in the United States. This is where the largest concentration of interest in the behavioral approach is found.
>
> *(p. 142)*

Even if patients cannot be cured, they may achieve "functional restoration." What this means in practice is that a person can, despite experiencing pain, resume some normal activities, including work. Merskey saw a danger in this way of thinking:

> Now, that fits nicely with the American belief that you should always cure yourself out of anything and overcome any obstacle. And that's an admirable belief, but it doesn't fit with the patient's real experience, which is that the pain can become intolerable for many people, though not for all. I'm not saying that some people don't get better, but many, many don't. But the insurance companies will line up to engage you to run these programs. And when the people finish the program, the insurance companies say, "Well, you dropped out of that program or you've graduated from it, so we don't need to pay you now." And there is . . . the motive power for a lot of America[n] pain clinic behavioral programs.
>
> *(p. 143)*

In other words, a person's "real experience" may be negated because of the pressure to reduce costs and to have patients resume employment when they have achieved functional restoration, regardless of experienced pain. Indirect support for this view comes from Vendrig (1999), who observed that "a change in the perceived disability status is the key element necessary to return patients with chronic back pain to work" (p. 217). Although functional restoration does not aim at denial of patient experience, the possibility for abuse remains.

Fordyce (1988) was critical of overextending the medical model of pain. If pain is always seen as a sign of injury or tissue damage, it can inadvertently contribute to needless disability, a result of admonitions to patients to rest or remain inactive beyond a period that would promote healing. What the medical model ignores is "the effects of prior experience and patient expectancies on the intensity of suffering and, accordingly, the intensity of pain or suffering behavior" (p. 282). He claimed that a behavioral approach reduces the ambiguity of treatment that "forces" patients "to determine whether healing had progressed enough to permit resumption of activity," in the face of medical "instruction" and "admonition," and substitutes for this ambiguity a "healing time [that] was defined by the physician" (p. 282). Whatever the merits of such regimentation, what is not removed in the process is the passivity of the patient in the face of physician and psychologist authority.

A critical problem with functional restoration lies in its very functionalism. Stam (2000) discussed the limitations of a functional approach to health, which he saw as being pervasive in biomedicine generally and in health psychology in particular. If one "considers 'healthy' the patient who has regained the ability to perform" (p. 278), one can foreclose personal, social, political, and ethical aspects of an individual's life and well-being. Functional restoration may result in coercive efforts to have an individual become productive again despite pain and with greater suffering as a result of functional, largely economic, understandings of well-being as the productive life.

Wailoo (2014) addressed the overarching political entanglements that behavior therapy implied, especially during the 1980s. During the Reagan years, there was a backlash against the earlier expansion of the terms of disability: "People claiming disabling pain embodied the problems of liberalism: a love of malingering and refusal of hard work, tolerance for welfare dependence, judicial gullibility, and extreme social indulgence" (p. 101). On the political level, there was a reversion to theories from before the 1960s: A 1984 "law stated that 'an individual's statements as to pain . . . shall not alone be conclusive evidence of disability . . . there must be medical signs and findings' " (p. 121). "Subjective pain . . . became a symbol of the dependence, the learned helplessness, and the growth of government that conservatives so detested" (Wailoo, p. 128). Taking these comments together with Merskey's, we see that economic and political force fields were present in the debates over the gate control theory, Merskey's operational definition, and Fordyce's behaviorism.

Critical perspectives

Constructing chronic pain

Weir Mitchell was thinking of anesthesia when he wrote his poem "The Death of Pain," but the sentiment applied to the sensation theory as well. If there are telephone line signals that produce pain, then there are clear ways to kill the pain, including nerve blocks, surgeries, and narcotic drugs. The promise of the sensation model is the death of pain. It carries this promise because its prototypical pain is acute. Where the model failed was with many types of chronic pain. With the challenges to Cartesian dualism in the mid-twentieth century came bad news. Melzack (1974) indicated the unrealistic fantasy that surrounds pain: "The idea of the ultimate panacea of *total* pain relief for *everyone* pervades our Western culture" (pp. 276–277; italics in the original). The new constructions reduced expectations. For many a patient, "the most effective therapy may be to teach them to live with their pain, to carry on productive lives in spite of it" (p. 277). This humbler goal is also implicit in behavioral approaches to pain. Fordyce, Roberts, and Sternbach (1985), in defending behavior therapy against its critics, disagreed with the notion that the end of such training is that patients are more stoical:

> The problem arises from confusing the hypothesis that pain *behaviors* can be learned and unlearned with the notion that *pain* can be learned and unlearned. Behavioral treatments for chronic pain are intended to reduce the *disability* associated with chronic pain problems.
>
> *(p. 120; italics in the original)*

Patients often do report less pain, "but decreased pain per se has never been a primary goal for these rehabilitation methods" (p. 121).

With these post-Cartesian constructions of pain, the emphasis shifted from acute to chronic pain, which had always been there (Hodgkiss, 1991). The new constructions admitted that chronic pain may not end. The critical questions here concern the meanings of "productive lives" and "functional restoration." If understood in terms of economic activity, this new humility can be coercive. Political and economic pressures to reduce expenditures on pain and disability had to reckon with the "bad news" that chronic pain may resist treatment. Constructions of pain from the 1960s on sought ways of reconciling people having persistent pain and resuming productive activity.

Body image and dualism

These three assaults on dualism and on real pain have had limited effect. As we will see with social representations of chronic pain, mind–body dualism remains a largely tacit assumption. As Jackson (2011) observes: "Most people continue to rather categorically oppose 'real' (organic, physical) pain to 'all-in-your-head' (imaginary, mental, emotional, or psychosomatic) pain" (p. 379). She cites Buchbinder (2010), who points out that such a dichotomy underlies the evaluation procedures of insurance companies and workers' compensation boards. Nevertheless, the three challenges to this dualism, albeit compromised, represented a shift in the construction of pain.

The gate control circuitry, the turn to pain as experience, and the shift of emphasis to behavior are all more true to experience than was the sensation theory, with its ringing bell. These innovations, however, all turn on the same conception of the body. Dualism is not surpassed, despite all best efforts; there is still a "category-mistake" (Ryle, 1951, p. 16). Pain is simply not a concept that can be put into parallel with anatomical concepts. While it remains for the next part of the book to address a meaningful way to categorize pain, here we raise the question of embodiment and of body image as a way of rethinking the issues raised in this chapter. Constructions of pain will always be dualist as long as the anatomical image of the body is their theoretical ground.

All three innovations implicitly recognize this dilemma, especially as they address the ways in which pain has emotional, motivational, cognitive, and social qualities. However, all three give a privileged status to the anatomical body image, especially its neurological activity. The nervous system remains the ground of them all and, in so being, these innovations, with the exception of Merskey's definition, make the error of misplaced concreteness. They take the experience of pain and place on the same plane concepts such as the nerve, the brain circuit, and anatomically verifiable tissue damage, which are products of natural scientific reflection. This grounding of pain in the abstract conforms to what the phenomenologist Alden L. Fisher (1957) saw as the scientific reconstruction of the lifeworld:

> The experience from which the science, properly so-called, then starts is no longer the immediately given of untampered-with experience, but an objectified or selectively abstracted experience. This is what is called the objectification process of science and refers properly to the fundamental scientific endeavor. But there is a second, equally important, which is the level of construction, or what amounts to a reconstruction, of the world.
>
> *(p. 148)*

Pain is reconstructed as, fundamentally, a neural reality. This abstraction infects even Merskey's operational definition, insofar as descriptions of pain are still in terms of the anatomical image of the body and not embodied subjectivity. The undoing of this abstraction is the work of the second half of this book.

Pain, illness, wounds, anxiety, and loneliness can alter the basic experience of human embodiment (Toombs, 1992). Then the body stands out objectively as a possession. This is the kind of experience at the root of the objectified body. The objectified body, the anatomical image of that objectified body in particular, is a powerful and important reconstruction of embodiment. It gives the gift of distance between the experiencing person and the disorder and pain of living; it creates boundaries between a person and those who would care and treat him or her. When a person is in a medical clinic, dualism renders invisible the personhood of the person. Only what is "objective" is available for scrutiny. Merskey's definition implicitly recognizes this dualism, in that no peering eyes can determine the truthfulness of the report of pain. The same happens with a behavioral approach, most dualistic of all, with its noninterference in the pain experience. The gate control theory, however, inserts these disparate phenomena onto the same circuit board.

It is significant that the three critiques we have examined came at the same time that the interdisciplinary pain clinic was growing as a cultural institution.

Is there a connection between these theories and the new clinics? Merskey and Spear advocated a monistic conception of pain but a dualist conception of the causality of pain. This odd position reflected real dilemmas in the treatment of pain, which led to the rise of pain clinics beginning in the 1950s. By and large, these centers recognized that purely biomedical treatments, especially of chronic pain, were insufficient, and they embraced a variety of nonmedical and psychological treatments as necessary. Pain escaped biomedicine, with its surgical and drug treatments. Pain was a mystery. Dualist assumptions underlie biomedicine, however, and what we find in these three attacks on Cartesianism in medicine is an effort to rethink the ground of medicine itself. We may ask: Does pain require a different conception of embodiment, one that avoids the inherent dichotomies found in the biomedical conception of the body?

Notes

1 This section drawn in part from Kugelmann (1997).

2 Implicit in Stengel's address was the notion that psychogenic pain occurs because the body that hurts is not simply the biologically understood body but the "lived body" (not a term that Stengel used, but in keeping with Schilder, whose work was used by Merleau-Ponty in his phenomenology of the body).

3 This is another instance of the category mistake that Merskey sought to avoid with his critique of "pain nerves." Suffering is a response of a person and involves the nervous system. A nervous system cannot suffer; it can only alter its electrical and chemical activity.

References

An interview with Patrick Wall (1925-2001). (2015). *The Physiology Society.* (Interview conducted 1999.) Available: http://www.physoc.org/oral-history-transcripts.

Anand, K.J.S., & Craig, K. D. (1996). New perspectives on the definition of pain. *Pain, 67,* 3–6.

Ayllon, T., & Michael, J. (1959). The psychiatric nurse as a behavioral engineer. *Journal of the Experimental Analysis of Behavior, 2,* 323–344.

Basbaum, A. (2011). Specificity versus patterning theory: Continuing the debate. *Pain Research Forum.* Retrieved from www.painresearchforum.org/forums/discussion/7347-specificity-versus-patterning-theory-continuing-debate

Beecher, H. K. (1959). *Measurement of subjective responses: Quantitative effects of drugs.* New York, NY: Oxford University Press.

Bendelow, G., & Williams, S. (1995). Pain and the mind-body dualism: A sociological approach. *Body & Society, 1,* 83–103.

Buchbinder, M. (2010). Giving an account of one's pain in the anthropological interview. *Culture, Medicine and Psychiatry, 34,* 108–131. http://dx.doi.org/10.1007/s11013-009-9162-2

Dallenbach, K. M. (1939). Pain: History and present status. *American Journal of Psychology, 52,* 331–347.

Devine, R., & Merskey, H. (1965). The description of pain in psychiatric and general medical patients. *Journal of Psychosomatic Research, 9,* 311–316.

Editorial. (1967). *Journal of Psychosomatic Research, 1,* 1–2.

Engel, G. L. (1959). "Psychogenic" pain and the pain-prone patient. *American Journal of Medicine, 26,* 899–918.

Engel, G. L. (1977). The need for a new medical model: A challenge for biomedicine. *Science, 196*, 129–136.

Fisher, A. L. (1957). Psychology or psychologies – A study in methodology. *Proceedings of the American Catholic Philosophical Association, 31*, 144–157.

Floor discussion: Operant conditioning. (1974). In J. J. Bonica (Ed.), *Advances in neurology, Volume 4: International Symposium on Pain* (pp. 591–593). New York, NY: Raven Press.

Fordyce, W. E. (1983). Behavior is behavior is. . . . *PsycCRITIQUES, 28*, 730. http://dx.doi.org/10.1037/022371

Fordyce, W. E. (1987). *American Psychologist, 42*, 312–315.

Fordyce, W. E. (1988). Pain and suffering: A reappraisal. *American Psychologist, 43*, 276–283.

Fordyce, W. E., Fowler, R. S., Lehmann, J. F., & DeLateur, B. J. (1968). Some implications of learning in problems of chronic pain. *Journal of Chronic Diseases, 21*, 179–190.

Fordyce, W. E., Roberts, A. H., & Sternbach, R. A. (1985). The behavioral management of chronic pain: A response to critics. *Pain, 22*, 113–125.

Gillies, V., Harden, A., Johnson, K., Reavey, P., Strange, V., & Willig, C. (2004). Women's collective constructions of embodied practices through memory work: Cartesian dualism in memories of sweating and pain. *British Journal of Social Psychology, 43*, 99–112.

Hebb, D. O. (1949). *The organization of behavior: A neuropsychological theory.* New York, NY: Wiley.

Hempel, C. G. (1965). Fundamentals of taxonomy. In *Aspects of scientific explanation and other essays in the philosophy of science* (pp. 137–154). New York, NY: Free Press.

Hodgkiss, A. D. (1991). Chronic pain in nineteenth-century British medical writings. *History of Psychiatry, 2*, 27–40. http://dx.doi.org/10.1177/0957154X9100200502

Honkasalo, M.-L. (2000). Chronic pain as a posture towards the world. *Scandinavian Journal of Psychology, 41*(3), 197–208.

Jackson, J. E. (1994). Chronic pain and the tension between the body as subject and object. In T. J. Csordas (Ed.), *Embodiment and experience: The existential ground of culture and self* (pp. 201–228). Cambridge, England: Cambridge University Press.

Jackson, J. E. (2011). Pain and bodies. In F. E. Mascia-Lees (Ed.), *A companion to the anthropology of the body and embodiment* (pp. 370–387). Malden, MA: Wiley-Blackwell.

Keeley, J. W., Morton, H. E., & Blashfeld, R. K. (2015). Classifications. In P. H. Blaney, R. F. Krueger, & T. Millon (Eds.), *Oxford textbook of psychopathology* (3rd ed., pp. 42–70). New York, NY: Oxford University Press.

Livingston, W. K. (1976). *Pain mechanisms: A physiological interpretation of causalgia and its related states.* New York, NY: Macmillan. (Original work published 1943)

Melzack, R. (1974). Psychological concepts and methods for the control of pain. In J. J. Bonica (Ed.), *Advances in neurology, Volume 4: International Symposium on Pain* (pp. 275–280). New York, NY: Raven Press.

Melzack, R., & Scott, T.J.H. (1957). The effects of early experience on the response to pain. *Journal of Comparative Physiology and Psychology, 50*, 155–161. http://dx.doi.org/10.1037/h0047770

Melzack, R., & Wall, P. D. (1965). Pain mechanisms: A new theory. *Science, 150*, 971–979.

Merskey, H. (1964). An investigation of pain in psychological illness. D. M. thesis, Oxford University, Oxford, England.

Merskey, H. (1965). The characteristics of persistent pain in psychological illness. *Journal of Psychosomatic Research, 9*, 291–298.

Merskey, H. (1966). Pain and the psychiatrist. *British Journal of Psychiatry, 112*, 637–638.

Merskey, H. (1982). Pain and behavior therapy. *PsycCRITIQUES, 27*, 1006. http://dx.doi.org/10.1037/020841

Merskey, H. (1983). Multimodel does not just mean behavioral. *PsycCRITIQUES, 28*, 730–731. http://dx.doi.org/10.1037/022372

Merskey, H. (1994). *Oral History Interview with Harold Merskey*, 8–9 October 1994 (Ms. Coll. no. 127.26), John C. Liebeskind History of Pain Collection, History & Special Collections Division, Louise M. Darling Biomedical Library, University of California, Los Angeles.

Merskey, H. (2000). History of psychoanalytic ideas concerning pain. In R. J. Gatchel & J. N. Weisberg (Eds.), *Personality characteristics of patients with pain* (pp. 25–35). Washington, DC: APA.

Merskey, H., Albe-Fessard, D. G., Bonica, J. J., Carmon, A., Dubner, R., Kerr, F.W.L., . . . Sunderland, S. (1979). Pain terms: A list with definitions and notes on usage. Recommended by the IASP Subcommittee on Taxonomy. *Pain, 6*, 249–252.

Merskey, H., & Spear, F. G. (1967). *Pain: Psychological and psychiatric aspects*. London, England: Baillière, Tindall & Cassell.

Oral History Interview with Ronald Melzack. (1993, October 16). Ms. Coll. no. 127.3, John C. Liebeskind History of Pain Collection, History & Special Collections Division, Louise M. Darling Biomedical Library, University of California, Los Angeles.

Perl, E. R., & Kruger, L. (1996). Nociception and pain: Evolution of concepts and observations. In L. Kruger (Ed.), *Pain and touch* (pp. 179–211). San Diego, CA: Academic Press.

Ryle, G. (1951). *The concept of mind*. London, England: Hutchinson's Universal Library.

Schilder, P. (1950). *The image and appearance of the human body*. New York, NY: International Universities Press.

Sherrington, C. S. (1900). Cutaneous sensations. In E. A. Schäfer (Ed.), *Textbook of physiology* (Vol. 2, pp. 920–1001). Edinburgh, Scotland: Pentland.

Slater, E. (1966). Pain and the psychiatrist: An open letter to Professor Stengel. *British Journal of Psychiatry, 112*, 329.

Stam, H. J. (2000). Theorizing health and illness: Functionalism, subjectivity and reflexivity. *Journal of Health Psychology, 5*, 273–283.

Stam, H. J. (2015). A critical history of health psychology and its relationship to biomedicine. In M. Murray (Ed.), *Critical health psychology* (2nd ed., pp. 15–30). New York, NY: Palgrave Macmillan.

Steger, J. C. (1981). Pain: Interface between the physiological and psychological. *PsycCRITIQUES, 26*, 943–944. http://dx.doi.org/10.1037/019872

Stengel, E. (1959). Classification of mental disorders. *Bulletin of the World Health Organization, 21*, 601–633.

Stengel, E. (1965). Pain and the psychiatrist. *British Journal of Psychiatry, 111*, 795–802.

Stengel, E. (1966). Pain and the psychiatrist: Reply from Professor Stengel. *British Journal of Psychiatry, 112*, 329–331.

Sternbach, R. A. (1981). Fundamentals of psychological methods in chronic pain. *Pain, 11*(Suppl. 1), 162.

Szasz, T. (1975). *Pain and pleasure: A study of bodily feelings* (2nd ed.). New York, NY: Basic Books. (Original work published 1957)

Toombs, S. K. (1992). *The meaning of illness: A phenomenological account of the different perspectives of physician and patient*. Dordrecht, Netherlands: Kluwer Academic.

Vendrig, A. A. (1999). Prognostic factors and treatment-related changes associated with return to work in the multimodal treatment of chronic back pain. *Journal of Behavioral Medicine, 22*, 217–232.

Wailoo, K. (2014). *Pain: A political history*. Baltimore, MD: Johns Hopkins University Press.

Wall, P. D. (1996). Comments after 30 years of the gate control theory. *Pain Forum, 5*, 12–22.

Wall, P. D., & Sweet, W. H. (1967). Temporary abolition of pain in man. *Science, 155*(3758), 108–109. http://dx.doi.org/10.1126/science.155.3758.108

PART II

Phenomenology and semiotics of pain

The first part of the book has explored, first of all, the construction of a narrow conception of acute pain as purely a sensation. This product of the sensation theory came in the wake of the development of anesthetics and analgesics, which promised the death of pain. These new drugs prepared the ground for this narrowing of the meaning of pain by finding their explanation and ground in the anatomical image of the body. With them, the abandoned body was realized in practice: the patient asleep as the knife exposed the disease hidden in the living cadaver. In thus affirming mind–body dualism, the way was paved for "real pain" and its shadowy twin: not-quite-real psychogenic and mental pain. The dualism at the basis of the sensation theory came under fire in the middle of the twentieth century from a number of directions without challenging the basis of the entire construction in the anatomical image of the body. However, the reconstructions described in the previous chapter rehabilitated psychogenic pain and dampened hopes for a death of pain. Chronic pain came into focus in the mid-twentieth century.

In the second part of the book, we turn to a phenomenological approach to pain. This approach suspends belief in the anatomical image of the body – not to disregard or deny it, but to look afresh at phenomena of pain from the point of view of embodied subjectivity. What emerges is an expanded conception of pain that encompasses the many ways that pain is experienced. This new conception goes beyond the definition proposed by Merskey in that it recovers some of what was lost in the debates over sensory pain. As experienced, pain comes in many forms. We begin with chronic pain, as it has defied the sensation theory in its persistence. Beyond the complexities of chronic pain, we shall see that psychological and moral pains are as much pain as chronic and acute physical pain. The phenomenological account is supplemented with a semiotic account of pain, which leads us to see that pain is, in addition to being something that afflicts us, a way of apprehending the world and ourselves. Pain happens with wounds to a person, and they occur in all spheres of life.

4

SOCIAL REPRESENTATIONS AND DISCOURSES OF CHRONIC PAIN

Chronic pain defies the assumptions of the sensation theory. Therefore, a consideration of it can help expand conceptions of pain, reconstructing it along phenomenological lines. This chapter examines the experience of chronic pain from three related perspectives: social representations, discourses, and a phenomenological analysis of the lifeworld of chronic pain. The social representations come from newspaper accounts of chronic pain from the early twentieth century to the end of the first decade of the twenty-first century, with the narratives and discourses from interviews with individuals in a pain management program. Finally, the chapter concludes with the appeals the narrators made for justice. In this way, chronic pain has an inherently moral aspect, and it can be said that these people were, among other things, experiencing moral pain.

Social representations of chronic pain

Social representation theory, initially developed by Serge Moscovici in social psychology, primarily addresses how societies absorb, reject, and modify expert knowledge, renewing common-sense knowledge in the process. Social representations do not simply popularize expert knowledge; they translate it into the common discourse of a society. They modify common-sense understanding through *anchoring*, the assimilation of new knowledge into the everyday sense of reality, and through *objectification*, in which metaphors, images, and explanations make the topic imaginable or quasi-perceivable (Moscovici, 2001, 2008).

Social representations of chronic pain reflect the translation of expert knowledge into common-sense knowledge, but in the assimilation of new knowledge, older ways of thinking about pain persist. Pain is hardly a new topic, and the religious, cultural, medical, and historical conceptions, narratives, images, discourses, and practices of pain remain. According to Encandela (1997), representations of chronic pain have been medicalized, reinforcing notions that pain is a sensation, with other aspects of pain obscured. An Irish study (MacNeela, Gibbons, McGuire, & Murphy, 2010) of social representations that physicians have of chronic lower back pain found that biomedical considerations dominated and were "largely silent on psychological and social aspects of this back pain" (p. 984). In verbal reports, representations "featured doubts over patient credibility" (p. 984). An Italian study (Nencini, Sarrica, Cancian, & Contarello, 2014) of representations of pain among healthcare professionals found that "pain that is not bridled by a clear cause-and-effect relationship evokes 'other' [than biomedical] forms of explanations, which draw on moral, ethical and evaluative dimensions, such as useful/useless, deserved/undeserved and benign/malign" (p. 926). These two studies narrowly focused on expert knowledge, not lay knowledge. What about in a broader social field? What follows are social representations of chronic pain drawn from newspaper accounts, largely but not exclusively from the United States.[1]

Before social representations of chronic pain

Moscoso (2012) claimed that chronic pain is a new category, a product of the twentieth century: "Its appearance coincided with the partial dissolution of what until that time had been called by the name of 'pain'" (p. 195), in part because the sensation theory accounted for acute pain but not pain that persists. At the same time, pain without ceasing was a part of the daily life of many, and Moscoso referred to Friedrich Engels and others who described the agonizing work and wretched living conditions of the poor: "The majority of people who have spent their lives gripped by pain find no place in the history of medicine" (p. 200). Chronic pain did not exist as a scientific object before the mid-twentieth century; as a result, there were no social representations of chronic pain, since social representations are based on scientific objects. Hodgkiss (1991) offered a somewhat different perspective. He found chronic pain widely discussed in nineteenth-century medicine, especially with complaints of pain that did not have corresponding lesions. Such "chronic pain without . . . lesion was a widely recognized and much discussed syndrome in the nineteenth century" (p. 30). Diagnoses proliferated, such as "neurosis" and "spinal irritation." Even though relentless pain received recognition, it did not form a single category like contemporary "chronic pain."

That late appearance – Witte (2014) dated its appearance into public discourse in the 1970s – is supported by newspaper reports. While there had been much discussion of chronic ailments, including pain, in American newspapers before the 1960s, there was no mention of chronic pain as a condition in itself. The term *chronic pain* was not unknown, but it was not the same thing as the chronic pain of the present day. As an example of early usage, here is an advertisement from 1905:

> Don't jump to conclusions and think, because you have suffered so long from chronic PAIN, that it is incurable. Whether you call it rheumatism, neuralgia, backache, earache, toothache, headache, a sprain, indigestion or

> some internal trouble, of which you don't rightly know the nature, the surest and most reliable relief and cure is HAMLINS WIZARD OIL.
>
> *("Don't Jump")*

The key phrase is "whether you call it." Many illnesses cause pain, and Wizard Oil kills it all, thus locating it in the line of Davis' Pain Killer, which Pernick (1985) described as the first remedy marketed specifically for pain. What we find with chronic pain in its social representations is that chronic pain has become an entity in its own right.

The beginnings of chronic pain as a distinct entity

The earliest reference to chronic pain as a disease entity I have found was in an article about U.S. President John F. Kennedy's personal physician, Janet G. Travell. Travell was an authority on muscle pain, and she is credited with helping JFK deal with chronic back pain, famously prescribing a rocking chair:

> More medical skills should be directed toward the relief of chronic pain, Dr. Janet G. Travell . . . declared here yesterday. She said that since her White House appointment she had received "a flood of letters" seeking her help in such relief. The appeals convinced her, she said, that "the alleviation of pain per se has not received the attention it deserves."
>
> *("Kennedy Doctor Widens Activity," 1961)*

However, the general public did not know the extent of Kennedy's pain or indeed much about his medical condition. He presented a picture of "vigor" to the world (see Altman & Purdum, 2002). Kennedy did not become, as he might have, the public face of chronic pain.

Older views of pain – the sensation theory and the distinction between organic and psychogenic pain – persisted into the 1960s (Boehm, 1966; Halberstam, 1967), even as the newer view began to appear. Jane E. Brody, a writer on health for the *New York Times*, wrote one of the first articles on chronic pain. Brody (1971) described a presentation by a Chinese acupuncturist who demonstrated what this treatment could and could not do for the relief of chronic pain. Significantly for social representations of chronic pain, a patient reported that her shoulder pain "did not respond to traditional methods of treatment" but did respond to acupuncture. This dichotomy between traditional (meaning medication and surgery) and nontraditional forms of treatment has been an important social representation.

Newspaper representations of chronic pain

The ways that newspaper articles contributed to the formation of the social representations of chronic pain differ. The *New York Times*, especially with science writers such as Brody and Daniel Goleman, who was also a psychologist, tended to disseminate expert knowledge to a broad public. The function of the articles was largely educational. Many of the *New York Times* articles mediated between the experts and the general public, and authoritative columnists wrote feature articles about pain. By contrast, in smaller newspapers, articles propagated social representations of chronic pain:

> The primary function of propagation . . . appears to be to organize and transform a theory into a whole which is compatible with the principles which establish the unity of the group. *Its second function is not to encourage a specific behaviour, but to prepare the group to behave in specific ways and to check that it does so, or to give it a meaning that it did not previously have.*
>
> *(Moscovici, 2008, p. 281; italics in the original)*

Propagation opens up new possibilities for thinking and acting for specific groups, which is why its appearance in community newspapers especially makes sense. At times, the writer ends the article with mention of a talk or other opportunity to learn more, and often the writer is a practitioner who lives in the local area.

The emergence of social representations of chronic pain

By the mid-1970s, one begins to find articles on chronic pain. A significant contribution to the representations was "Solving the Mystery of Pain" by Laurence Cherry (1977), who wrote extensively on medicine and psychology. Cherry introduced innovations in the science of pain and the International Association for the Study of Pain to readers. His article provides a compendium of the social representations of chronic pain.

Pain as a warning bell

Ordinarily, pain is a "warning bell," a phrase that objectifies pain in an imaginable term, because a warning bell is a simple electronic device that is part of the commonsense world. In chronic pain, "the body's helpful warning bell has itself become a threat to well-being" (Cherry, 1977, p. SM12). The warning bell misfires, and that is chronic pain. Cherry connected this image of the bell with the nineteenth-century innovation of the telephone and the isolation of "pain nerves." Pain nerves were "like tiny telephone wires, connected to a switchboard like [a] mechanism in the brain" (p. SM12). This older representation of pain had its limits, and Cherry addressed the flaw in an analogy: It "almost totally ignored the role of emotion" (p. SM12). In place of the telephone analogy, Cherry introduced the gate control model of pain.

The gate

Cherry's presentation of the gate control theory – what he called the "spinal-gate theory" (p. SM13) – is a central representation of pain in the article. The account develops the electrical circuit metaphor for the nervous system. This account of codes, cables, network, and gateway gave form to the mechanisms of chronic pain by assimilating it to everyday experiences of wiring and electronic communication. The technological imagery also suggested potential know-how that would enable treatment of the pain. Cherry's representation of the gate control theory drew upon common-sense images of pain as an "it" that attacks a person. Not surprisingly, the image of the gate conforms to the common sense that alleviation of pain is the chief thing to know about it.

Pain relief through techniques old and new

Cherry's article addressed, as did many, the promise of new treatment and explanations for tried-and-true techniques to relieve pain. Older remedies, "such as hot-water bottles" (p. SM13) work because they stimulate "the large fibers and [suppress] the small fibers that produce pain" (p. SM13) by means of the gate control system. Gate control theory also explained innovative techniques, including acupuncture. The reader is nowhere presented in this article with explanations of acupuncture in terms of the movements of *chi*, the cornerstone of traditional Chinese medicine. What happens is that the needles "shut the pain gate" (p. SM13). The opening and closing of gates and electrical circuits was part of the everyday lifeworld, but for most readers of the *Times*, *chi* would not have been common sense. Continuing along the electrical circuit analogy, Cherry discussed "electric pain suppressors" that were inspired, at least in part, by the gate control theory, and Cherry quoted the neurosurgeon C. Norman Shealy, who had developed a "dorsal column stimulator" that would deliver electrical impulses to the spine to relieve pain. "These impulses abolish the pain signals," Cherry explains, although he admitted that "no one is sure exactly why or how these devices work" (p. SM50). Such caution characterizes the entire article, even the presentation of the gate control theory which, he cautioned, "remains controversial" (p. SM13). Moscovici (2008) called accounts with this kind of hesitation in the dissemination of representations "diffusion," because the author does not impose a view on the readers. Such tentativeness plays a role in social representations of chronic pain, especially in controversies over the place of drugs and surgery in the treatment of pain.

Pain control with chemicals made by the nervous system

Part of the discourse surrounding innovations in conceptions of pain had to do with the discoveries of endogenous opioids, with Cherry mentioning enkephalin and the endorphins. He depicted how these chemicals acting in the nervous system can prevent pain. The promise was a potential end to "the long quest for a safe and effective pain-reliever" (p. SM53).

Psychological aspects of pain

Cherry concluded his article with the role of emotions and other psychological aspects of pain. Pain is something that can be lessened by patient activity; pain is not simply a warning bell. Cherry discussed biofeedback in terms of muscle relaxation. Hypnosis is mentioned, but without an explanation of how it might work. Most of this section of the article is devoted to Fordyce's "conditioning techniques" and to an example of their use. The program sought to wean patients from analgesics and substitute other ways of coping with pain. In addition to pain relief coming from muscle relaxation and mental exercises, patients were given new ways to look at the treatment of pain, and these ways played a role in what was under debate in the social representations of pain: "The goal of this strategy is obvious: to end any psychological benefit the patient may derive from their pain" (p. SM53). There is a sense, in these newspaper accounts, that many patients resisted knowledge of the role of psychological factors in chronic pain, as that seemed to deny pain's reality. They held on to representations that they are passive in the face of pain and that relief is to come primarily from drugs and surgery. This battle played itself out over the decades.

Social representations of chronic pain, 1980–2014

Not surprisingly, most of the newspaper accounts addressed the nature of chronic pain and how to treat it. They typically began and concluded with stories of individual patients, stories that personalized the condition. Some articles reported on the sufferings of public figures, such as a Supreme Court judge, actors, and athletes dealing with chronic pain. By 1993, chronic pain was named without comment, suggesting that it had become a taken-for-granted medical condition and was not controversial or unknown. Letters to the editor typically argued a point, such as the undertreatment of pain or the addictive nature of painkillers, thereby touching nodal points in the social representations of chronic pain. What follows is a summary of significant representations of chronic pain from newspaper accounts; these are indicated by double quotation marks.[2]

Social representations of the disorder

"Chronic pain" is a legitimate medical condition; it is "real pain." The prototype of pain remains "acute pain," which is patently real in this field of significations, short-lived, a "warning bell" of something wrong, and a symptom of disease or the result of surgery. The accounts stress "physical causes" of chronic pain in specific locations in the body, especially in the back, as such causes remain the gold standard of reality. However, "emotional causes" and complications of chronic pain are also factors, with the doubt, lurking in the wings, that it is "all in your head." Compounding the emotional distress is "the invisibility of chronic pain," and complaints surface that physicians and others do not "believe" that the pain exists – hence, pain sufferers insist on the reality of chronic pain.

An important representation was the assertion that "all pain can be relieved." Also represented was an opposing claim: Chronic pain, articles acknowledged, often cannot be eliminated entirely, unlike acute pain. The phrase "learn to live with it" was vilified, which no one cited actually advocated. Experts admonished readers that while not all chronic pain could be cured, it was possible to reduce pain and lead a full life despite it. "Leading a full life" had its contrast in "drug dependence" and fears of "addiction."

Basic to the social representations of chronic pain was the "mind–body dichotomy" in terms of causes. This dichotomy of physical and emotional (psychological) causes of the pain leads to the social representations of treatment.

Social representations of treatment

The fundamental representations of a mind–body dichotomy appeared in the talk of treatment options. The two most general representations were "medical" and "nonmedical" forms of treatment. The assumption was that "real pain" responds to medical treatment, meaning drugs and surgery. Chronic pain, with emotional causes compounding physical causes, does not always respond to drugs and treatment, and as a "last resort," patients turn to pain clinics that often specialize in nonmedical treatment. Although "pain clinics" had been around for some years, they began to appear in stories about chronic pain in 1977, and during the 1980s they were repeatedly introduced, suggesting that they had not yet taken root in common sense.

Medical treatment was problematic in a number of ways. On the one hand, there was consistent concern about how chronic pain was "undertreated" and that physicians did not seem to understand the gravity of the pain that patients presented. On the other hand, there was anxiety over "doctor hopping" and "overprescription" and with misguided drug treatment leading to "addiction." Addiction was one of the most prominent nodes in this network of representations and was internally conflicted; it was argued that opioid use by pain patients did not lead to addiction, and yet there were fears that it did. Representations of opioid addiction are older than those of chronic pain, and there were active efforts to separate the two. Stories described how some physicians were being prosecuted for too generously prescribing painkillers. Occasionally, stories dealt with the use of illegal drugs for pain, but more dealt with the use and abuse of prescription drugs such as OxyContin. The tension within this field seems in part to be generated by the attitude that "real pain requires drug treatment." The treatment of emotionally caused chronic pain can lead to the overuse of drugs, with addiction as a consequence. Herbert Burkholz, an American novelist and for a while a speechwriter for a commissioner of the U.S. Food and Drug Administration, wrote one of the many introductory articles on chronic pain. Burkholz (1987) likened a chronic pain unit at a hospital as having "a marked resemblance to a drug rehabilitation program or a group therapy clinic" (p. SMA32). In presenting a program to wean patients from narcotics, Burkholz also discussed the body's ability to produce its own narcotics, with the hope that they could be synthesized; he concluded with eyes to the future: "The goal, then, is a world in which all pain can be controlled, inexpensively, effectively and without the risk of drug addiction. It is a goal that is finally in reach" (p. SM35). The promise that pain can be "conquered" remains at the root of the social representations of chronic pain. Representations of chronic pain seem to have been selectively assimilated into common sense to keep the hope for the "death of pain" alive.

Around the topic of nonmedical treatment swarmed a number of representations. Individual treatments were periodically introduced over the decades, including acupuncture, relaxation, biofeedback, and electrical devices. Advocates of these measures had to ward off the "it's all in your head" accusation about chronic pain while supporting the notion that emotions can be a cause or a consequence of prolonged pain. As time passed, explanations of these techniques drew increasingly on "brain activity" rather than "gate control." In fact, the "brain" is likely to replace the "gate," "emotions," and the "mind" as an explanation. Arguments included the view that "drugs do not work" and that surgery can sometimes be ineffectual for chronic pain. Fears of addiction played into the promotion of nonmedical techniques.

The plot line of the social representations

The social representations were not only a set of terms that mediated expert knowledge and everyday knowledge; there was an implicit plot or master narrative. The key term here was "mystery." Chronic pain is a mystery, and many of the accounts hinted at, hoped for, and anticipated a solution to the mystery. They offered hope of an ultimate cure at the same time that they stressed the need to accommodate the tenacity of chronic pain.

Discourses of chronic pain

Recurrent themes in the study of chronic pain include patient struggles with the invisibility of pain and the felt need to prove its reality (Clarke & Iphofen, 2008), difficulties that social representations of pain echo. The question of the reality of chronic pain affects individual identity (Ojala et al., 2015). The totalizing quality of chronic pain – the way it consumes a life – and its deceptive invisibility and problematic causality can lead to "narratological distress" (Lavie-Ajayi, Almog, & Krumer-Nevo, 2012), with individuals struggling between a narrative of leading a normal life and one in which the narrator is disabled. Kirkham, Smith, and Havsteen-Franklin (2015) addressed the invisibility of pain by studying drawings that pain patients created of their pain. One theme that emerged in the paintings was the threatening, foreign, and violent sense of pain in the lives of these individuals. To explore these and other themes, we turn to the experience of chronic pain.

Experiencing chronic pain[3]

Because the reality of the pain was an issue for the participants, as it often is with chronic pain (Jackson, 1992; Walker, Sofaer, & Holloway, 2006), as we have seen already in its social representations, I begin with the terms used by the participants in a qualitative study that I conducted (Kugelmann, 1999). I interviewed individuals (and some couples) who were in an inpatient pain management program. I was not a member of the staff. The patients were primarily working-class men and women, aged between 20 and 50, White, Black, and Hispanic, from Texas. Most of the participants had suffered work-related injuries to their necks and backs. The terms in which they described their pain defined it as a discursive object. Then, we turn from discursive polarities to the lifeworld of pain revealed through these polarities. This analysis centered upon the torment of having to inhabit the intolerable and how, simultaneously, people construct pain.

Finally, after these considerations of the terms in which pain is described, the study turns to the act of "saying" pain, a turn influenced by Levinas (1991), for whom speech is first of all an address (the "Saying") by someone to someone, the basis for speech meaning something (the "Said"). The participants were not simply informing me; they were making claims on me. What they were saying, not surprisingly, had the form of complaints or – to use an archaic word – "plaints" – laments and protests. Complaint was the genre of these interviews. Following Cowan (1984), genres are "fundamental orientation[s] toward reality . . . perspectives on life that indicate the kind of response being called for by a particular work" (p. 7). In addition to complaints, there was something tragic in the narratives. For Cowan (2003), tragedy is not a "perspective" but an opening to the abyss, the groundlessness of human existence, which in Western literature often comes as a Fall and the opening up of "the realm of suffering – loss, fragmentation, pain" (Cowan, 1984, p. 9). Individual descriptions of living with chronic pain thus drew upon forms of telling that have deep cultural roots.

We can recast the challenges of chronic pain to identity in terms of the lived body. While the phenomenological underpinnings of this approach will be developed in the following chapters, it is important to state that chronic pain is a mode of being in the world. As Merleau-Ponty (1962) stated, there are many "ways for consciousness to be consciousness" (p. 124). Pain is one of them, as Honkasalo (2000) affirmed: "Pain is a bodily attitude, a position and posture taken in the world, towards the world. A posture of longing for the lost past" (p. 203). Honkasalo asked the critical question: "What is chronic pain about?" (p. 204). Its "aboutness" is not thereby an explicit intentionality, because pain comes unbidden.

In being about the lived body, pain is also about lived time. In a general way, "being in pain is an embodied judgment about the finitude of human existence – the experience of chronic pain in its cruelty and destructiveness is perhaps . . . one of the closest to the edges of life itself" (Honkasalo, 2000, p. 205). More explicitly, Honkasalo found that "people in pain concretely hold on to their previous worlds – a relation that in so many ways is reminiscent of a love relationship. The grasp is so tight that there is no space for release, for bereavement or sorrow" (p. 205). It is holding together a disrupted world, a finding of an earlier phenomenological study as well: People in chronic pain "struggle . . . to be true to one's past, to sustain it in the present and to project it into the future" (Murphy & Fischer, 1983, p. 294). We collectively and individually construct pain along the same lines we construct love and grief. Chronic pain, even in its physicality, resonates on emotional and moral levels of existence as well.

Discursive polarities of chronic pain

The stories the participants told had many contexts, the foremost being the fact that they told their stories in an institutional context. They were students as well as patients, for they were being taught a particular understanding of pain. The pain management program taught a biopsychosocial model of pain that emphasized the importance of active participation, not simply compliance, in treatment. Hence, in addition to occupational therapy, exercise programs, and lessons in "body mechanics," patients also participated in biofeedback, guided imagery training, stress management, and often individual psychotherapy. As Saris (1995) described it, "a narrative of a chronic condition is not simply a story of personal experience. It is, rather, deeply embedded within various institutional structures that influence its production as a story" (pp. 39–40). Many of the participants were being introduced for the first time to the effects of stress upon their pain, and their stories reflected their agreement or disagreement with this explanation. In addition to the specific institutional setting, there were larger cultural categories that shaped the telling of pain. As Honkasalo (2000) stated: "People's 'own' everyday life meanings are embedded in biomedical theories and explanations, and vice versa. They together shape a meaning structure resembling a beaded necklace: medical and lay explanations follow each other forming a meaningful pattern" (p. 204). In what follows, semantic polarities that the participants employed show how pain is socially constructed in both agreement and disagreement with biomedical and biopsychosocial models of medicine.

As we have seen with its social representations, chronic pain has had its very existence disputed, and the real and the unreal became the ultimate polarity in the interviews. The nature of pain was under constant negotiation, especially around issues of "responsibility for one's condition" and the possibility for "stigma and demoralization" (Jackson, 1992, p. 138). Slade, Molloy, and Keating (2009) observed:

> Stigma arises from external sources such as health care professionals, family and friends, the community, government agencies and insurance companies, and from other sufferers. Stigma can also arise from within, with sufferers experiencing guilt and blaming themselves for their pain.
>
> *(p. 147)*

Eccleston, Williams, and Stainton Rogers (1997) delineated conflicts within the "web of blame, responsibility and identity," which turn on "the meaning of chronic pain in the construction of identity" (p. 708). The problems of pain's reality and of responsibility arise because chronic pain defies Western categories, challenging and simultaneously affirming the dualities that define biomedicine (Kirmayer, 1988).

Discursive polarities are ways of describing pain, responding to pain, and assuming attitudes toward pain, in either/or terms. These terms tend to be taken for granted regardless of the speaker's attitude toward them. Some of the polarities bespeak a biomedical or a biopsychosocial medical narrative. Other polarities arise from popular American culture. As in much of the history of pain over the past century, *real* in the interviews meant *body*, although thought was acknowledged to be an active power. Throughout the interviews, pain implied passivity. Being active meant doing things to lessen pain. Activity went beyond simple compliance with medical advice; indeed, participants typically held that compliance was a form of passivity. Activity meant what they could do: physical exercise, dietary changes, and avoidance of medication or surgery. *Mind* meant initiative and self-determination; *body* implied passivity and conformity to biomedical treatment.

Stress and relaxation

A polarity of stress and relaxation was ubiquitous in the interviews. *Stress* has become a catchall explanatory term in popular as well as learned culture. The interviewees learned that stress affects pain, and they were taught means to alleviate stress. The discursive polarity of stress and relaxation was inseparable from the educative means used to instill it. Stress explained the effects of emotions and interpersonal relations on pain. One patient, a part-time preacher, stated: "What causes the pain to increase is stress. . . . I've seen it happen, me and my wife was coming to a . . . little argument, and a little stress would come on, and my knee would start throbbing." He emphasized that he had learned in the pain management program that stress causes an increase in pain. Relaxation reduces stress and pain:

> It stresses you out when they [his son] start arguing with you. So, I told him, "I'm not gonna get mad. I'm gonna stay in a relaxed state, but I'm gonna tell you this, you do it again and you're grounded."

Instead of getting angry, he practiced the relaxation technique he learned in biofeedback training. What is distinctive about this discourse is how it interprets interpersonal conflicts in engineering terms. The effect of another person is to alter pressure or tension, felt as tight muscles and other disturbances. Then, various means are available to alter the felt tightness. The discourse of stress can configure difficulties in interpersonal relations in terms of felt tension, which explains increases and decreases in levels of pain.

This polarity reduced diverse pain-provoking incidents to a common denominator. As the part-time preacher observed: "Tempers, tension, stress, anything like that, even financial problems, money problems, all that will cause stress, stress leads to pain." Physical strain also causes stress. A construction worker reported:

> I used to work all day and it'd never bother me, and now you can't even go for about an hour and I'm being sore. . . . Today it was just too sore to . . . putting up too much stress today.

Stress discourse postulates a mechanism whereby anything increases bodily tension and thus pain.

In conformity with the pain management program's position, interviewees tended to present relaxation as a safer method than, or as an adjunct to, self-medication with drugs and alcohol. As the part-time preacher described his understanding:

> You might get relaxed by the pill, but it stresses you out. . . . Everybody's been asking me all afternoon, what's wrong with me? Because I was on the pills. See, if I'd have gone ahead and done the biofeedback today, I'd have been a whole lot more alert.

Relaxation is a vague term, so it is important to discuss exactly what practices were involved. They consisted of listening to audiotapes of music or natural sounds, such as the ocean; meditative practices of quieting the mind; prayer; guided imagery; and biofeedback. While these practices (with the exception of biofeedback) are time-honored means of reckoning with suffering, as Foucault (1972) argued, two statements can differ radically from each other, even though semantically they say the same thing. To say that meditation is a means of responding to pain means one thing in Christian or Hindu spirituality and quite another in biopsychosocial medicine. In religious traditions, one can suffer pain for purposes of atonement or detachment; in the stress–relaxation polarity, pain is a disvalue to be managed.

This polarity presents pain as a problem to be solved. *Stressed out* meant being irrational, not using instrumental reason. A food-service worker recounted how her neck pain worsened when she had conflict with her sister:

> I just couldn't, the stress just couldn't from that moment of finding out that my child was gone and that my sister was behind it was really, just sent me, it took me a long time to calm down enough to even think about being rational.

Being rational meant having her emotions under control. These experiences link pain with emotion, and they contrast it to instrumental reason. A school cafeteria worker put the case this way:

> And it's very stressful . . . you have to deal with all your emotions constantly, because they interfere. Well, me and my husband argued . . . and I didn't stop crying till 2, and I then slowed down till I started talking to the counselor

> here and I started back up. . . . Because my emotions had overruled so much, that they had caused me so much pain now, to tighten the muscles.

Emotions are irrational, and they make muscles tense, cause pain, and hinder progress. The specific object of this polarity of stress is muscle tension. Cultural practices from earlier times are introduced as drug and alcohol substitutes in an effort to lessen the stress in muscles surrounding painful parts of the body.

Some patients said that learning to relax gave them some measure of control over pain. The part-time preacher put it in clearly dualistic terms:

> You can let [pain] bother you to the point where it will drive you crazy. You got to learn to take control over the pain, because actually, your pain is just part of your body, and if your spirit can take over the physical part of it, the physical part can't win.

Control over pain means release from pain, or it means not being overwhelmed by pain. Two participants, a substance abuse counselor and a veterinary worker, were involved in twelve-step programs, and they saw similarities between their relationships to pain and to alcohol. In both cases, "it" had control, and their lives were in self-destructive cycles. The veterinary worker stated what she had learned about pain:

> You control it. It's up to you. You choose it or you don't. It's kind of like being an alcoholic, you've got to get down as far as you go. You've got to hit your bottom, as they said in AA, which I did to get here and choose either to get better or die.

She claimed that she was no longer helpless and that pain was something she could influence. The polarity of stress and relaxation, in brief, takes up in an instrumental way the polarity of mind and body.

Physical and emotional pain

A second polarity involved physical and emotional pain. Interviewees clearly distinguished the two. The part-time preacher described difficulties he had had with getting a definitive diagnosis for his back pain:

> I go through this period probably for the first month of not knowing what's wrong with my back. . . . Well, nobody's found out what's wrong with me yet, so here we are. We're back in this emotional pain as well as physical pain.

His emotional pain was the anguish over his ignorance of the cause of pain and of the disorder pain introduced into his family's life. Even when the two pains were differentiated, they were related. A young construction worker stated that he knew how to deal with physical pain because he had been through other difficult times: "So me being through all that I had before this, no physical pain, but I've been through a lot of emotional pain that I know life's got to keep on going." The two pains were distinguished by their causes and by their temporal sequence: The physical pain in these stories always preceded emotional pain. This sequence was important, signifying the legitimacy of the patients' pain.

What brings the two together are the common ways to cope with them: drugs, alcohol, emotional outbursts, biofeedback, and so on. What also brings them together are the ways in which interpersonal conflict can exacerbate them. For the food-service worker, stories about her workplace, about her family, and about her quest for a diagnosis all centered on how the empathy or callousness of others affected her pain. Social isolation and the indifference of others worsened her pain. A warehouse worker described how, after surgery for back pain, he had to face the news that his brother-in-law had been murdered: "My wife, she's really taking that hard. That's another added thing. I think stress kind of brings on your pain a little, a little." The pain of the surgery, the residual pain in his back, and the pain of the loss are all pain.

Because the participants had no definitive medical explanation for their pain, they had no legitimized account that would have resolved the ambiguity between physical and emotional pain. The ambiguous character of pain in the interviews affords a glimpse through a crack in sedimented categories of the real. For the interviewees, this ambiguity could not be sustained, because pain discourse is simultaneously medical, legal, and financial (workers' compensation, Social Security, etc. are not extraneous factors). The warehouse worker's guarded repetition that "stress kind of brings on your pain a little, a little" needs to be understood in the context of his having filed a claim for disability assistance. To admit more would, in his own eyes, discredit his claim because it would mean that he really is not in pain (see Wailoo, 2014). The discourse on emotional and physical pain is significant as the site of conflict over legitimacy of suffering, continued financial support, and legal action against corporations and governments. The contemporary construction of pain cannot be abstracted from these considerations. Patients interpret their very sensations in light of the economically and politically codetermined nature of pain.

Positive and negative thinking

Closely related to the polarities of stress and relaxation and of physical and emotional pain was a negative–positive thinking polarity. In it, a self-defeating way of thinking was pitted against recipes for success, highlighting ways in which a person can be active against pain, because the polarity claims that attitude and mood can be willfully manipulated. The strategy for its deployment is the relief of pain through the control of one's attitude toward it. As the part-time preacher said: "Any time that I think negative, I'm stressed out, I'm not relaxed, I'm in pain. But if I think positive, then I'm more relaxed, and I'm ready to go." Positive thinking frees him from, whereas negative thinking keeps him trapped within, the circle of pain. In one statement, he brought together all the polarities discussed so far:

> To me, pain is physical and emotional on a person. And the only way to relieve yourself of pain is first of all, think positive, OK. Don't ever think negative. Think positive. OK, second of all, keep yourself out of stressful situations. And as far as your physical pain, learn the positions that you can get in that will make it a little bit less.

This discourse directs attention to a possible mobilization of personal abilities in the face of their disintegration. Positive thinking entails self-assertion, claiming that I can do something against pain, that thought and feeling can be harnessed to overcome pain.

The young construction worker described his approach to dealing with pain:

> There are two aspects that you can sit there and look at, the positive side and the negative side, which I'm pretty much of a positive thinker. . . . And now, I'm hurt and I can't do the things I was doing, but I don't get so down that I can't still live it, there's a couple of times that I just felt like giving up, and but if you give up you have nothing, no hope, no nothing, you don't have no backbone.

Negative thinking signifies weak character – someone who gives in to strong feelings. The polarity of positive and negative thinking points to the close relationship between pain and emotions, such as grief, depression, and despair.

One expression of this discourse of positive thinking is the notion of being "strong minded." Strong-minded people are self-reliant, do not express much emotion, and do not want to be dependent on others. They "deal with" pain because "it's a part of me," as the assembly line worker said. Overt expression of emotion can be a sign of weakness, and others might take advantage of it. The young construction worker said that he had learned to be strong minded in prison, where any display of soft feeling was an exploitable weakness. In this discourse, pain is weakness, because pain is failure to master one's feelings.

This polarity articulates how interviewees respond to being hemmed in by pain-imposed limitations. The part-time preacher observed:

> Pain can destroy a person. It can destroy your family, destroy everything you've ever tried to accomplish. I thought, OK, I'm never going to be able to work, I'm never going to be able to do this, never able to do that. Negative sayings, OK. I think a person needs to think positive about it, not negatively.

This statement depicts the devastation that occurs when pain constricts a person, and it identifies these constrictions as negative, thereby indicating that there is an active stance to take, one within one's own grasp – positive thinking.

One finds oneself at a turning point, where one can choose the negative or the positive.

One strategy of this polarity is to redefine chronic pain in spiritual terms, a not-unlikely possibility, insofar as "positive thinking" originated within American Protestantism and its secularization (Meyer, 1980). While none of the patients expected a miraculous cure through the power of positive thinking, those that spoke of pain in these terms asserted that pain was, in some degree, in their own hands. So while the polarity of positive and negative thinking reasserts the dichotomy of spirit and matter and the ultimate control of matter by spirit, it also – and more significantly – claimed that pain is not simply a matter of sensing and feeling but also a matter of thinking. In addition to the pragmatics of positive thinking was an assertion about the nature of pain.

Spiritual aspects of positive thinking touched on a person's reasons to "go on." Positive thinking, in one sense, means having the determination to live despite pain. Positive thinking reinterprets the negative in positive terms, as if life events could have, somewhat arbitrarily, positive or negative meanings. In fact, within the polarity, the value assigned is a matter of one's will. This discursive polarity draws on the ideology of willpower, deeply rooted in our self-help culture (Kugelmann, 2013).

Pain invisible and visible

The most frequently employed polarity was that between the invisibility and the visibility of pain. Pain's invisibility made it difficult to understand. "People comprehend what they can see," the assembly line worker noted. Pain is, in this way, not independent of its expression and of the persuasive abilities of the person claiming to be in pain. These considerations of the visibility and invisibility of pain help determine the construction of chronic pain.

The invisibility of pain differentiates it from observable forms of suffering. The veterinary worker stated:

> This is an invisible illness. . . . Somebody in a wheelchair or somebody who's got a disease, cancer or broken bones, you know something's wrong. . . . And a lot of people: "Oh, you're not hurt that bad," because they can't see it.

The lack of obvious evidence for the pain had social consequences for this woman: "It hurts when your family can't make allowances, because it's invisible to them." When pain persists after the scars have healed or time has passed, patients find themselves isolated in their pain. Moreover, the invisibility of pain in part stems from a belief that pain should not survive the original injury, that it should be acute.

The participants were frustrated when told that an X-ray or other visualization of the body showed nothing amiss, especially when financial benefits or continued treatment hinged on medical evidence. As the young construction worker stated:

> That's what I got to get through to these psychologists and to this doctor . . . so that they'll believe me and start looking at it as a severe pain instead of

> something that's in my head or some unexplained reason. I need to make them try to believe me and that's the hard part.

Difficulties with interpersonal validation of the reality of pain placed many of these patients in the dilemma of "needing" pain in order to prove that they are in pain. Precisely because it is invisible, everyone involved seeks to reveal it.

However, pain is also visible. Pain shows itself as behavior and expression. The assembly line worker described how her children and her fiancé would see that she was hurting and not let her do some household chore that she habitually had done. The veterinary worker's boyfriend, who had studied massage, could feel her pain when he massaged her back:

> I could feel when she was hurting real bad because her whole body sent signals to me when I was touching her, and you could feel – and then there were certain points in her body like, right at the base of her spine where there was a big knot.

Other interviewees pointed to similar experiences, some of which happened when the patient was attempting to hide all expression of pain. Pain's visibility is its expression so that it is a matter of self-display. In this polarity, only showing oneself can show pain to others. Visible pain renders a person vulnerable, exposed in his or her weakness.

Because of the ambiguous visibility of pain, the question of belief surfaced. Interviewees complained about not being believed when they claimed that they were in pain. However, the question of belief went both ways, and many interviewees did not believe what physicians or others told them about their condition, especially when their own experience contradicted medical authority. Affirmation of their own accounts, especially by medical authorities, afforded emotional relief.

Often, belief had important medical, legal, and economic consequences. The food-service worker spoke of her dilemma in trying to get workers' compensation, especially after her supervisor failed initially to report her accident:

> They sent me for different tests just to see and they also sent me to an orthopedic doctor at that time and he didn't think that there was anything seriously wrong. And when I went for my workman's comp, my attorney would never listen to me because physically he saw a healthy person.

Pain is a social, legal, political, and economic, as well as medical, condition. But because of what counts as objective in the contemporary order of things, pain that outlasts the mending of bones and tissue is subject to disbelief.

A polarity of mind and body

The aforementioned polarities reflect contemporary distinctions and divisions between mind and body. These differences correspond to those Kirmayer (1988) describes: mind means activity, body passivity. Body also means real, and mind means unreal or imaginary. The conjunction of passivity and reality of the body occurs because *body* can be offered as evidence of the claim of pain. While the existence of the pain management program indicates that there is some acknowledgment of the social dimension of pain, the repeated claims of the participants to be taken seriously show that they experience pain as primarily their private responsibility, whose existence they must prove – with medical and legal denotations of *prove*. This tension between the activity of mind and its ties with unreality seems to threaten to make individual initiatives futile. The polarity of mind and body finds expression in the insistence by participants that they be believed. For the participants, *belief* was the issue because they felt isolated within themselves. *Mind* in this context means isolation, a shadow side of individuality: Something private needs to be made public.

Constructing chronic pain in contemporary discourse

In light of these polarities, how was pain constructed in the interviews? Pain is something that must be produced as an objective entity; pain must be brought forth as evidence. It is not self-evident. Pain must also be produced in the sense that it must be continually sustained. Finally, given the character of what counts as evidence and the manner in which pain exists as an object of contemporary discourse, pain must be produced in the sense of being endlessly evoked in the dialogue between those who claim its presence and those who compensate for it and treat it. These discursive practices have their institutional setting: pain management programs, designed to manage pain – that is, make it less costly economically and socially. Pain is produced within an economic, medical, and legal web, a web that seeks an equilibrium of efficient functioning.

Pain, in these discursive polarities that define it, is a private possession of the individual that must be produced in an objective manner if it is to be a social reality. The speaker stands as the one responsible for the production of pain. Pain is defined in such a way as to affirm and negate, simultaneously, the dichotomies that define it.

The lifeworld of chronic pain

The body as lived is not simply the passive object of an active mind. Phenomenologically speaking, the body as body-subject is the "I can" (Merleau-Ponty, 1962, p. 137). However, as pain often shows, there are times when "I cannot." That inability to move, to act, also constitutes me as a body-subject. The limits of ability are also those of one's situation. In severe pain, the world is "unmade" (Scarry, 1985, p. 42). Pain is "world-destroying" (Good, 1994, p. 121); pain can create a "biographical disruption" (Bury, 1982, p. 167). Such destruction or disruption occurs in the world understood phenomenologically, the lifeworld, which is one's lived situation. At the same time, it is not inevitable that a serious illness be lived as disruptive (Delbene, 2011; Williams, 2000). While there is no doubting the destructive power of intense or prolonged pain, other things may be more important to an individual than the pain. There is, moreover, a way in which pain is world making. From a phenomenological point of view, pain is an affliction within existence. The very undergoing of pain, the handling of pain, the expressions of pain, and the descriptions of pain construct pain and, in so doing, construct the world. It may not be a desirable world.

Pain and existence: loss and grief

Chronic pain leaves no aspect of life untouched. In pain, one can "lose it." The veterinary worker felt abandoned when a physician said, "Here, take this pill" and offered nothing else. She felt lost to drugs, to drink, to physical and social isolation and immobility, to depression and despair. The expression *lose it* expresses aspects of the life situations of the participants. The truck driver's wife stated that her husband "will never be pain free," and she described the difficult adjustment to and the limitations of his injury and pain, saying, "It's a grief process." With protracted pain, one loses one's taken-for-granted way of life. That world is right there, separated from one by an invisible boundary. One's familiar self and world have died. The young construction worker stated:

> It's heartbreaking, you have your heart set on doing something and you've always done it and you can't do it, it's kind of like when you lose one of your loved ones, it's not really that bad but it's something that you do love and it's not there no more.

Pain and grief share a great deal.

A number of the interviewees severely restricted their activities because walking or being in a car hurt them or because they feared that activity would exacerbate their pain. Some interviewees found themselves mourning losses of activities and occupations. The limits that pain placed on activities included possibilities for being with loved ones. The truck driver stated: "I can't do some things I would really love to do with [my son]. . . . I can't really get out there and teach him the things I would like to teach him."

The grief of pain was sometimes described in terms of depression. While depression – with all the vagaries of the term – and chronic pain – with similar ambiguities – can be seen as separate syndromes, it is closer to the sense of the interviews to see them as complementary modalities of the same phenomenon (Lerman et al., 2015). Pain signifies loss of a customary world and of an ability to do things. The loss is both of the self and of the world. In pain, one loses aspects of the world because one can no longer engage the world in those ways. As we say, "grief hurts," so we could also say, "hurt grieves."

In these narratives came descriptions of things that brought enjoyment. Just as pain signified emotional pain as well as physical pain, pleasure, too, did not have a univocal sense. Because of this range of meaning of the terms, these descriptions focused on the place of love in the patients' lives. Being with others in enjoyable activities countered the isolation of pain. The relationship between pleasure and pain in these accounts again emphasizes the connection between grief and pain: Enjoyment and love counter pain.

Pain and being in place

"Pain causes you limitations." Pain is a way of being in the world or, more specifically, a way of "being-in-place" (Casey, 1993, p. xv). The place of pain is, of course, the body, but it is the body-in-place – that is, within a historical, social, political, and economic field. The young construction worker expressed his defiant isolation: "You're going to have to learn how to cope with the pain and the best way to do it is just yourself." The electronics worker spoke of trying to sleep her pain away with painkillers: "And it wasn't that I was eating that much [that she gained weight], it was that I was sleeping that much." Pain had pulled its noose tightly.

Pain is an existential situation. It was described as a confinement, symbolically as a prison (see Olivier, 2007). The school bus driver/teacher spoke about being housebound by pain: "Other than my doctor's appointments, I had to stay home. I felt like I was in prison so to speak, however that feels, very depressing." The electronics worker described her situation: "It's like I'm being slowly tortured and it's like there, it's like everything I need is somewhere, somewhere behind some door." The place of pain was also depicted as a kind of homelessness. Two of the women feared actual homelessness because of loss of earning power, coupled with abandonment by family or spouse or employer. Pain is a kind of "homelessness," because it casts one out of one's everyday world, bereft of security. Beset with such anxieties, the veterinary worker consented to an abortion, which she later regretted. She had feared not being able to take care of a baby and said her boyfriend was "adamant" about the abortion. The electronics worker also spoke about fears of homelessness, of being "thrown back" into poverty and crime. She feared that she would not be able to work because of her pain and that she would not qualify for disability benefits. Pain, which limits self-reliance, places one in the boundary situation of homelessness: not having a place.

A historical and social precondition for these existential locations is the social and economic requirement for adults to be self-reliant. For the participants, chronic pain implied indigence. Both prison and homelessness, as names for the place of pain, have a common element: In both instances, the person is cut off from the possibility of dwelling, of being at home. The part-time preacher stated that his pain had surrounded him: "I was in the center. Now I'm on the outside. I'm on the outside and pain is on the inside. And the pain that I had, I was on the middle before." Pain as the perimeter of existential place is significant. It suggests that pain itself is a boundary, a limitation.

Pain presents itself as more of a non-place, because the place of pain cannot be inhabited. Participants described themselves as restless. That restlessness, or inability to maintain any position for a great length of time, was the primary embodied way that they constructed pain. As several of the interviewees stated, in describing how they try to have a positive attitude: "I don't dwell on things" like the losses that pain entails. This attitude of not-dwelling is not simply a volition that one freely accepts or not: It presents itself as intrinsic to pain itself, such that the taking up of an attitude such as *I will dwell on pain* would be the radical departure. In this light, recall the observation of Bradley (1888) that restlessness is the "chief effect of pain" (p. 14).

The electronics worker recounted a dream she had that put her in her grandmother's house. What stands out is a gathering of a community as the occasion of the end of pain:

> Ever since I started this pain, I haven't had dreams like I used to. I dreamt of this house. It used to be my grandmother's, at least the living room. It's like I walk inside and there's this coffin way at the end and I know it's me. And I go towards it real slow and it's like everywhere I turn, everybody's in white. But I keep on going to this coffin, and it's my arm in the coffin. So, everybody like started clapping and celebrating and it was like, you know, I felt it. I felt that happiness in me. I felt it. I'm not in pain no more you know.

This dream located the end of pain in a "living room," a place to dwell and to celebrate. The end of pain was an end to mourning, putting the loss to rest.

Pain attunes one, according to these accounts, to the gaps and fissures of existence, and chronic pain constructs the world by showing how radically contingent and incomplete it is, how each person dances on the edge of a precipice. In this is pain's tragic dimension. Pain attunes one to the abyss. One does not dwell in pain – there is no living room there – for one restlessly seeks relief, seeks being brought back to common ground. Hence, the practices discussed previously, particularly positive thinking and biofeedback, appear now as assertions of dwelling: Thinking achieves distance from the immediate situation, transforming actuality through perception of possibilities. Biofeedback seeks a "disappearance" of the body (Leder, 1990, p. 25) so that the lived body can resume its career as the background of everyday tasks.

The polarities discussed earlier assume that the dualism of *mind* and *body* can be overcome: Positive thinking and relaxation, for example, might make the body conform to the mind. Chronic pain invites the dark thought that dualism is existential. It is, again, a tragic sense of things: There is something wrong with me, with the cosmos. Gadamer (1996) quotes the Greek physician Alkmaion:

> "We human beings must die because we have not learnt to connect the end with the beginning again and this is something we can never accomplish." This is a genuinely disturbing observation for it tells us that it is not something in particular that we lack, but rather everything.
>
> *(p. 97)*

Pain constructs and deconstructs the everyday world, showing its contingency.

A cry for justice

A recent phenomenological study found that questions of justice were endemic in the lives of people with chronic pain, especially as they feel misunderstood and ignored (McParland, Eccleston, Osborn, & Hezeltine, 2011). In a similar vein, for Good (1994): "A great many anthropological studies of illness have shown that sickness is universally experienced as . . . a rupture of the moral order" (p. 134). These issues – the meaning of suffering and hopes for deliverance from it – organized the "saying," the activity of the participants telling me their stories. I was addressed by them, called by them to witness their pain. First, the act of saying took the form of a complaint. These complaints were, first of all, plaints or laments about their situations. Second, they were accusations, at times made against specific individuals or institutions, at other times against "the way things are." Third, they were calls for rectification. Some participants spoke as dependents of service institutions. Yet they also spoke as people beholding firsthand the human inability to "connect the end with the beginning" and nevertheless hoping to do so.

The genre of the narratives was that of complaint: the statement of a grievance, of grief, wrong, loss, and suffering. Older views understood pain to exist because the cosmos itself was flawed. The flaw has been interpreted in a myriad of ways: Judeo-Christian, Platonist, Hindu, Buddhist (Illich, 1976). This perception of pain occurred in the interviews, often expressed in the ambiguities of the word *wrong*. Pain is something wrong. Pain was tied to injustice, not only for actual injuries done but also with pleas to be heard. The polarities through which the participants expressed themselves – of mind and body, of negative and positive, of stress and its relief – are culturally available ways of lamenting, of complaining, of crying out for justice. Buchbinder (2010), developing this genre of complaint in interviews about chronic pain, observed that the complaint interrupts the narrative and seeks another end:

> The medical anthropological research interview, as a particular genre of complaint, makes a claim for certain retributive ethical judgments and thus privileges certain types of accounts. . . . A sort of narrative interruption can occur when narrators choose to highlight "one pain or another pain."
>
> *(p. 126)*

The complaints I heard were situation specific, especially as the economic security of many of the participants was at stake, as were insurance benefits, with participants under pressure to reduce drug usage and use nonmedical forms of treatment.

Complaints had a tragic tone. The food-service worker described the responses of her supervisors to her fall and injury:

> But they never once said, "Do you have to go to the doctor?" I told them I was in pain. I was in tears because I couldn't sit, I couldn't hardly stand, I couldn't hardly walk, I was like, "Please, acknowledge that I'm not well."

This woman felt wronged: In the first place, there was something wrong medically that caused pain, and pain should not be. In the second place, she felt wronged by her employers and her physician, who did not acknowledge or assist her. Throughout the interviews, most of the patients were not merely describing, they were pleading. While a few were literally plaintiffs in a legal sense, all were plaintiffs in existential terms. Complaints were not necessarily directed against anyone. They were instead directed primarily against the way that they found themselves. The complaints assert that, in one sense, pain is "unnatural": that to be a human being, to live a human life, is incompatible with being in pain. This implicit assertion did not stem from a desire for perpetual anesthesia but from a felt sense of what a good life is. The complaints were not only about present pain or past wrongs but also about aborted futures, as the electronics worker indicated: "I was going for my bachelor's degree and I had two good offers before I got injured." She could not return to her former occupation, and she felt that despite her hard climb out of poverty, she was being thrown back into it, through no fault of her own. At other times, the complaint was lodged in terms of an archaic discourse, that of harmony or of natural balance (Gadamer, 1996), as was the food-service worker's:

> And I mean, I was like, God, I hope you're never on the end of the rope similar to yours because "what goes around comes around." And one of these days, somebody's going to do you the same way that you're doing your own employees.

To cause pain, or to fail to respond to the pain of another, violates the nature of things, according to this statement. It asserts that pain is an evil.

Blame is implied in the etymology of "pain" (*poena*, "penalty"), so that pain is punishment for some wrong done. Pain, blame, and responsibility have wider significance, however (Eccleston et al., 1997). Others were to blame for much of the pain, and some participants felt that they themselves were to blame. In other instances, some felt that they were being blamed for having pain. While scapegoating did not surface in the interviews, it was an implicit threat felt by many participants, especially in the insistence with which they claimed that their pain arose from an accident and was not their fault. Much of the pleading about the anatomical site of pain must be understood as the participants pleading their case.

The question of responsibility thus arose. The substance abuse counselor took responsibility for his pain in these terms: "What's true is you've let your goddamn health go in the toilet, and you're trying to blame it on somebody else." The young construction worker ambivalently blamed his boss and fate for his accident: "Our boss was pushing us, you know, I figure it was just my day to get hurt." The medical assistant expressed ambivalence: "He [my husband] doesn't *blame* me for it, you know, but at times I blame myself for it, but I'll sit there and tell him and he'll get upset with me for doing that." The electronics worker emphatically blamed the company she worked for: "They should at least say, 'Yes, we're to blame.' But I haven't heard from anybody. I mean, it's just like what am I complaining about."

In the logic of these complaints, pain isolates a person by severing relationships with a community. When pain exists, when this rupture of community occurs, then someone or something is responsible for it. This is the thesis, to which there is an antithesis: It was just an accident. However, even then, a wrong must be made right. With blame comes the question of payment for pain. This is not simply seeking to exploit pain as a secondary gain. Rather, it indicates that pain demands an equivalent in someone else's substance. These demands, which might appear to be malingering or a refusal to take responsibility, address the primary sense of something being amiss in pain. The school cafeteria worker asserted that "the only thing I regret is that I was never said, 'I'm sorry.' These kids never came up to me and said, 'I apologize,' but I just want the pain to stop. I want my life back." An apology would not give her her life back, would not connect the end with the beginning, but it would "set things straight" between her and the kids. Payment here means, at the very least, an apology, a response to the sufferer's complaint: "Apology does not blindly affirm the self, but already appeals to the Other. It is the primordial phenomenon of reason, in its insurmountable bipolarity" (Levinas, 1969, p. 252).

Recalling that these cries to rectify wrongs take place in a pain management program, I conclude that these stories of complaint resemble legal proceedings. Some of the participants had received or anticipated a legal judgment regarding their status as disabled. Their desire that physicians take them seriously only reinforced my sense that the narratives had a quasi-legal form. It is as if the interviewees were pleading their cases before someone who would act as a witness. They spoke from the no-man's-land of "homelessness" or "prison" of pain, in a context that involved both determination of proof of pain and release from pain.

Critical reflections

Depictions of chronic pain were similar in the social representations and the interviews: In both, the question of the reality of the pain surfaced in conflicts about forms of treatment, especially when nonmedical treatment threatened participants' sense of the reality of their pain. In both were polarities of mind and body. In addition, the interviews showed the liminal world of chronic pain (pain as not being able to dwell, such that in pain the sufferer is imprisoned or homeless). Finally, in hearing the complaints, we unfolded some of what the social representations were about in everyday communication. In both the social representations and the interviews, two contradictions appear: First, the polarities present pain as private property, a meaning amplified by the sense of imprisonment, in which the person in pain feels trapped with a private reality that often cannot be brought forth with public evidence. Pain as revelatory of a broken world contradicts the sense of it as private and personal. The homelessness and imprisonment to which the not-dwelling of pain can be compared is not a private reality but an existential one. Insofar as we all share in pain, what pain reveals, it reveals to all. The participants in this study experienced pain primarily as their private property, with little cash value. In their isolation, the painfulness of pain becomes amplified. Pain, however, is not private: It connects us with a broken world.

The second contradiction that emerged was the contradiction between representations of the invisibility of pain – that is, the difficulties that people in pain have of producing evidence that they are in pain – and the demand for justice that the participants insisted upon. The setting for the interviews – the pain management program – provided the courtroom, as it were, for these cries. There, the participants assumed, evidence would have to be physical: an X-ray, a diagnosis, an assessment. Nevertheless, the premise of these trials militated against acceptable evidence being brought forth. Pain became visible, however, in another way in responding to the complaint, by entering into the narrative, at the very least, and witnessing the pain that shows itself there.

A non-Cartesian duality finds expression in the complaints about pain. The genre of the complaint, the laments and accusations of these stories, affirm that for these people, pain was first of all a moral question. This moral question shows us the duality involved: *I am in pain; I should not be in pain. Other dualities, between my current state and what preceded it, between myself and the others who inflicted pain on me, flow from this one.*

Pain, like love, is a cultural construction. Like love, it can tear one's world apart, and like love, especially unrequited love, it entails a hope to have one's case heard. Like its analogue, it involves laments. Unlike love, we construct chronic pain in calls for justice, in complaints against the wrongs that tore apart everyday life. In this regard, chronic pain is moral pain.

Notes

1 Three newspaper databases were used in this study, with 150 articles used as data for a qualitative analysis using a phenomenological approach: *Chronicling America* (http://chroniclingamerica.loc.gov/) for the earliest articles; *ProQuest Historical Newspapers: The New York Times*, which extends from the 1850s to the present (most of the material came from this source, especially for the period 1960–2014); and *LexisNexisAcademic* for the period after 2000.

2 These social representations are drawn from a qualitative research analysis of 150 newspaper articles from 1837 to 2014. Most of them date from after 1977.

3 This section and the next draw upon Kugelmann (1999).

References

Altman, L. K., & Purdum, T. S. (2002, November 17). In J. F. K. file, hidden illness, pain and pills. *New York Times*, p. 1.

Boehm, G. (1966, September 11). Aspirin doesn't cure any disease. *New York Times*, p. 304.

Bradley, F. H. (1888). On pleasure, pain, desire and volition. *Mind, 13*, 1–36.

Brody, J. E. (1971, December 15). Acupuncture demonstrated at medical parlay here. *New York Times*, p. 26.

Buchbinder, M. (2010). Giving an account of one's pain in the anthropological interview. *Culture, Medicine and Psychiatry, 34*, 108–131. http://dx.doi.org/10.1007/s11013-009-9162-2

Burkholz, H. (1987, September 27). Pain: Solving the mystery. *New York Times*, pp. SMA16–19, SMA32, SMA34–35.

Bury, M. (1982). Chronic illness as biographical disruption. *Sociology of Health and Illness, 4*, 167–182.

Casey, E. S. (1993). *Getting back into place: Toward a renewed understanding of the place-world.* Bloomington: Indiana University Press.

Cherry, L. (1977, January 30). Solving the mystery of pain. *New York Times*, pp. SM12–13, SM50–53.

Clarke, K. A., & Iphofen, R. (2008). A phenomenological hermeneutic study into unseen chronic pain. *British Journal of Nursing, 17*, 658–663.

Cowan, L. (1984). Introduction: The comic terrain. In L. Cowan (Ed.), *The terrain of comedy* (pp. 1–18). Dallas, TX: Dallas Institute of Humanities and Culture.

Cowan, L. (2003). Introduction: The tragic abyss. In G. Arbery (Ed.), *The tragic abyss* (pp. 1–22). Dallas, TX: Dallas Institute of Humanities and Culture.

Delbene, R. (2011). Patients' narratives of chronic illnesses and the notion of biographical disruption. *Communication & Medicine, 8*, 17–27.

Don't jump. (1905, January 21). *Daily Press*, p. 4. Retrieved from http://chroniclingamerica.loc.gov/

Eccleston, C., Williams, A. C., & Stainton Rogers, W. (1997). Patients' and professionals' understandings of the causes of chronic pain: Blame, responsibility and identity protection. *Social Science & Medicine, 45*, 699–709.

Encandela, J. A. (1997). Social construction of pain and aging: Individual artfulness within interpretive structures. *Symbolic Interaction, 20*, 251–273.

Foucault, M. (1972). *The archaeology of knowledge* (A.M.S. Smith, Trans.). New York, NY: Harper & Row.

Gadamer, H. G. (1996). *The enigma of health.* Palo Alto, CA: Stanford University Press.

Good, B. (1994). *Medicine, rationality and experience: An anthropological perspective.* Cambridge, England: Cambridge University Press.

Halberstam, M. (1967, February 5). Patients who make the doctor feverish. *New York Times*, pp. SM18–19, SM74–76.

Hodgkiss, A. D. (1991). Chronic pain in nineteenth-century British medical writings. *History of Psychiatry, 2*, 27–40. http://dx.doi.org/10.1177/0957154X9100200502

Honkasalo, M.-L. (2000). Chronic pain as a posture towards the world. *Scandinavian Journal of Psychology, 41*(3), 197–208.

Illich, I. (1976). *Medical nemesis: The expropriation of health.* New York, NY: Pantheon.

Jackson, J. E. (1992). "After a while no one believes you": Real and unreal pain. In M.-J. D. V. Good, P. E. Brodwin, B. G. Good, & A. Kleinman (Eds.), *Pain as human experience: An anthropological perspective* (pp. 138–167). Berkeley: University of California Press.

Kennedy doctor widens activity. (1961, April 20). *New York Times*, p. 23, 44.

Kirkham, J. A., Smith, J. A., & Havsteen-Franklin, D. (2015). Painting pain: An interpretative phenomenological analysis of representations of living with chronic pain. *Health Psychology, 34*(4), 398–406.

Kirmayer, L. J. (1988). Mind and body as metaphors: Hidden values in biomedicine. In M. Lock & D. R. Gordon (Eds.), *Biomedicine examined* (pp. 57–93). Dordrecht, Netherlands: Kluwer.

Kugelmann, R. (1999). Complaining about chronic pain. *Social Science & Medicine, 49*, 1663–1676.

Kugelmann, R. (2013). Willpower. *Theory & Psychology, 23*, 479–498.

Lavie-Ajayi, M., Almog, N., & Krumer-Nevo, M. (2012). Chronic pain as a narratological distress: A phenomenological study. *Chronic Illness, 8*, 192–200.

Leder, D. (1990). *The absent body.* Chicago, IL: University of Chicago Press.

Lerman, S. F., Rudich, Z., Brill, S., Shalev, H., & Shahar, G. (2015). Longitudinal associations between depression, anxiety, pain, and pain-related disability in chronic pain patients. *Psychosomatic Medicine, 77*, 333–341.

Levinas, E. (1969). *Totality and infinity* (A. Lingis, Trans.). Pittsburgh, PA: Duquesne University Press.

Levinas, E. (1991). *Otherwise than being or beyond essence* (A. Lingis, Trans.). Dordrecht, Netherlands: Kluwer Academic.

MacNeela, P., Gibbons, A., McGuire, B., & Murphy, A. (2010). "We need to get you focused": General practitioners' representations of chronic low back pain patients. *Qualitative Health Research, 20*(7), 977–986.

McParland, J. L., Eccleston, C., Osborn, M., & Hezeltine, L. (2011). It's not fair: An Interpretative Phenomenological Analysis of discourses of justice and fairness in chronic pain. *Health: An Interdisciplinary Journal for the Social Study of Health, Illness and Medicine, 15*, 459–474.

Merleau-Ponty, M. (1962). *Phenomenology of perception* (C. Smith, Trans.). New York, NY: Humanities Press.

Meyer, D. (1980). *The positive thinkers.* New York, NY: Pantheon.

Moscoso, J. (2012). *Pain: A cultural history* (S. Thomas & P. House, Trans.). New York, NY: Palgrave Macmillan.

Moscovici, S. (2001). The phenomenon of social representations. In G. Duveen (Ed.), *Social representations: Explorations in social psychology* (pp. 18–77). New York: New York University Press.

Moscovici, S. (2008). *Psychoanalysis: Its image and its public.* Malden, MA: Polity.

Murphy, M. A., & Fischer, C. T. (1983). Styles of living with low back injury: The continuity dimension. *Social Science & Medicine, 17*, 291–297.

Nencini, A., Sarrica, M., Cancian, R., & Contarello, A. (2014). Pain as social representation: A study with Italian health professionals involved in the 'Hospital and District without Pain' project. *Health Promotion International, 30*(4), 919–928. http://dx.doi.org/10.1093/heapro/dau027

Ojala, T., Häkkinen, A., Karppinen, J., Sipil, K., Suutama, T., & Piirainen, A. (2015). Chronic pain affects the whole person – A phenomenological study. *Disability and Rehabilitation, 37*, 363–371.

Olivier, A. (2007). *Being in pain.* Frankfurt, Germany: Lang.

Pernick, M. S. (1985). *A calculus of suffering: Pain, professionalism, and anesthesia in nineteenth-century America.* New York, NY: Columbia University Press.

Saris, A. J. (1995). Telling stories: Life histories, illness narratives, and institutional landscapes. *Culture, Medicine and Psychiatry, 19*, 39–72.

Scarry, E. (1985). *The body in pain: The making and unmaking of the world.* New York, NY: Oxford University Press.

Slade, S. C., Molloy, E., & Keating, J. L. (2009). Stigma experienced by people with nonspecific chronic low back pain: A qualitative study. *Pain Medicine, 10*, 143–154. http://dx.doi.org/10.1111/j.1526-4637.2008.00540.x

Wailoo, K. (2014). *Pain: A political history.* Baltimore, MD: Johns Hopkins University Press.

Walker, J. M., Sofaer, B., & Holloway, I. M. (2006). The experience of chronic back pain: Accounts of loss in those seeking help from pain clinics. *European Journal of Pain, 10*, 199–207.

Williams, S. (2000). Chronic illness as biographical disruption or biographical disruption as chronic illness? Reflections on a core concept. *Sociology of Health and Illness, 22*, 40–67.

Witte, W. (2014). The emergence of chronic pain: Phantom limbs, subjective experience and pain management in post-war West Germany. In R. Boddice (Ed.), *Pain and emotion in modern history* (pp. 90–110). New York, NY: Palgrave Macmillan.

5

CONSTRUCTING PSYCHOLOGICAL PAIN

Real and imaginary; physical and mental; sensory and emotional: Dualities still haunt pain today. This situation is not simply an intellectual problem; it reflects being with pain, for as the anthropologist Jean E. Jackson (2011) writes: "Pain is the quintessential symbol of disorder" (p. 372). Could it be that there is in pain something that resists efforts to order it, as there is with eros, injustice, and death? Pain is not only a symbol of disorder; it exceeds order.

In this chapter, we turn to psychological pain as described in everyday situations. We have seen that chronic pain resonates in multiple regions of existence, from the bodily to the social and the moral. What about everyday experiences of pain? What do people say? What is pain in the vernacular? We examine in particular a type of pain often denied existence as pain: psychological or emotional pain. Is the "suffering of psychological pain, hurt, and distress resulting from separation, divorce, death and other losses" (Staats, Hekmat, & Staats, 1996, p. 194) a way that individuals construct real pain? The answer to this question depends on a turn away from the anatomical image of the body as *the* ground upon which we construct pain. If, in place of wounds to the anatomized body, the abandoned body, we substitute the lived body, then psychological pain (with its unfortunate connotation of dualism) is pain.

In the previous chapter, we considered chronic pain, an example of pain in a medical context. Now we step away from medicine. Eccleston (2013) went in this direction in a study of transitory, minor, and relatively unproblematic pain. He identified two aspects of everyday pain that go beyond professional preoccupation with its sensory qualities. First, pain, in addition to being private and personal, is also "a social and communicative event" (p. 47). As a type of social occurrence, pain connects and separates people, calling forth from others aid or scorn, among other things. Second, "pain functions to interrupt other concerns or mental preoccupations and to motivate escape or avoidance" (p. 47). Pain disrupts the individual's world, provoking efforts to restore or renew that world.

Psychological and physical pain[1]

In a phenomenological study of everyday pain, a question commonly arose when my students and I asked people to describe a time when they were in pain: *Do you mean physical pain or emotional pain?* The reply was that it did not matter. Whatever they felt to be pain was pain. The resulting descriptions of pain, regardless of their alleged cause (a broken bone or a broken heart), had similar forms and plots. These narratives involved a "fall" out of a shared world to a place of hurt. There emerged a desire for something else, which proved to be the key moment.

The reality of psychological pain

That pain was not only sensory or physical was a commonplace of the nineteenth century. French psychiatry at the time viewed psychological pain (*la douleur morale*) as a cause of some mental illness, especially melancholia (Masson & Muirheid-Delacroix, 2014). While psychological pain suffered eclipse for many years, Masson and Muirheid-Delacroix wrote that Anglophone authors had rediscovered *la douleur morale*, with labels such as "moral pain, psychache, psychological pain, emotional pain, psychic pain, mental pain" (p. 142). Others have argued for "social pain" (MacDonald & Leary, 2005) and psychological pain (Mee et al., 2006). Recent studies using neurological imaging techniques found similar brain circuits active in psychological as in physical pain. Masson and Muirheid-Delacroix suggest that the imaging techniques extend the visibility of pain, furthering the medical gaze (Foucault, 1973) – that is, imaging technology appears to make subjective experience objectively available. Biro (2014) contends that pain can be caused "*solely* by psychological damage" (italics in the original), such as from "betrayal, grief or depression" (p. 54). He offers an expanded definition of pain as "the aversive feeling of injury to one's person and the threat of further, potentially more serious injury" (p. 61). By shifting the location of the wound from the anatomical image of the body to the person, this definition advances a reconstruction of pain. Everyday psychological pain is just as "real" as pain from tissue damage. It was important for my study that it was outside any medical settings, which assume the anatomical image of the body.

An analysis of the narratives identified existential dichotomies and challenges to them. Everyday pain showed itself as an activity of a person, an action nevertheless characterized by passivity – that is, as a suffering of something rather than actively doing something. Experiencing pain as an "it" manifests this passivity, as "it" is the active agent, not "me." This experience of pain as an "it" and as not-me shapes the kind of performance that pain is, whether identified as psychological or physical. The term *performance* captures the scripted character of pain in social settings. I use *performance* instead of *behavior*, which is too entailed in behaviorist thought and misses the fact that pain is done by a person, not an organism.

Pain as a performance is not all of the story: Pain is an *it*, yet pain is *I*; pain isolates me from the social world, yet pain exposes me, leaves me vulnerable, throbbing with every insult and look of scorn. This I/it is like another whom I cannot face, afflicting me prior to any decision regarding it, belonging to a domain that also includes love, justice, and death, as did chronic pain. As with chronic pain, there is a felt loss and a hunger for something absent.

Similarities between psychological and physical pain

The narratives of psychological and physical pain had similar plots. They began with a felt sense of being wounded, they altered the existential world, they disabled, and they isolated.

Felt sense

Psychological pain, like physical pain, was embodied. The narrators described a felt sense (Gendlin, 1978–1979) in specific bodily locations: "I felt such pain – it was and still is this emptiness in my heart. My heart physically hurts, not like a heart attack, but more like a burning sensation." Most frequently, psychological pain was in the chest, yet other locations were affected: an "uneasy feeling in my stomach," "on my shoulders," "a dumbstruck feeling like you would get after someone punches you real hard in the stomach." This finding is in line with the International Association for the Study of Pain (IASP) definition that pain is "described in terms of such [tissue] damage." However, the felt sense refers to the lived body or perhaps to Szasz's (1957/1975) notion that pain is "the affect referring to ego-bodily orientation" (p. 77). This "ego-bodily orientation" is not the "useful, functional, prosaic body" of biomedicine; it is the "symbolic or poetic weight" (Merleau-Ponty, 1969, p. 83) of the flesh. Psychological pain in other studies was often described in terms of these same bodily locations and at times as the worst pain a person had ever felt, worse than that of a broken leg (Mee et al., 2006, p. 682).

The narrators described pain in other ways: "During my times of emotional hurt my heart felt like it was frozen and I couldn't breathe. My eyes hurt so much from crying that my head hurt and I had no appetite." "Emotional hurt" meant that some interpersonal event "caused" the pain; this pain expressed in crying led to a "physical hurt." Crying, grimacing, hiding in one's room, seeking help, and so on – what is called pain behavior – constituted performances of pain. A felt sense radiated outward from the original site of pain: The exhaustion of tears and the loss of appetite were also felt and felt as pain. Temporal rhythms, felt intensity, and the waxing and waning of feeling happened in both types of pain. Gündel and Tölle (2005), differentiating sensory and emotional aspects of pain, show how the distinction may be sometimes impossible to make.

Disability

Pain afflicts and can disable any activity, including walking, grasping, swallowing, remembering, and thinking. One's lived body becomes figural and obtrusive (Leder, 1990) in pain. Injuries to the hand, leg, and back leave sufferers at least temporarily immobilized and attentive to their wounds. Pain can be peripheral or central to personal projects:

> I have horrible neck and shoulder pain [after a car wreck] . . . It makes it very hard to study comfortably without having some neck support. My pain . . . can make me cranky or not able to concentrate.

Pain demands attention (Eccleston & Crombez, 1999), which is potentially disabling.

What participants called psychological pain likewise disabled: "I didn't do anything, I just sat still and stared in front of me." Loss of a love made remembering difficult: "It hurts to think of good times because you miss those times. It hurts even worse to think of bad times because you see the way things really were." The pain of grief made thinking a burden: "I could not bear the thought of never seeing her again. Sometimes, I still feel pain when I think about the funeral, or her absence." Note that here the metaphor of "bearing" was also a felt sense. Metaphor connects and distinguishes types of pain. This disabling also applied to memory: "Remembering brings it back, but it is not nearly as strong now." Pain made remembering burdensome. Some participants protected themselves by not thinking, as others did by not moving a painful organ. Narratives spoke of an inability to sleep, to get out of bed, and to move on to other relationships, and they also described loss of energy and composure.

Pain as affliction

Pain is not only something that happened, an "it"; it is also an activity. Psychological and physical pains were ambiguous as to whether they were ways the narrators attended to the pain or ways they painfully attended to something: "It was a very intense and radiating pain. I tried to distract myself from it . . . but my mind kept going back to the pain." In another instance: "The pain . . . was a horrible constricting feeling I felt in my heart because I was misunderstood by my family." This pain was both that of rejection and of an inability to deal with a difficult social situation. Pain could also be a performance of undergoing, an "it" that assailed: "It didn't hurt that much until . . . I stood up. Sharp pain filled my back, I couldn't breathe, my legs were numb with pain." Characterizing these afflictions were "double sensations" (Merleau-Ponty, 1962, p. 95) of the lived body: The body was nearly simultaneously object (the thing felt) and subject (the act of feeling). Pain was reflexive – hence the ambiguity of *I hurt* and *it hurts.* Particular to pain's double sensibility was a twofold recoiling: from the situation that caused or prolonged the pain and from the pain itself.

If pain intended anything, it intended affliction: a suffering or undergoing. Two instances illustrated this thesis; the first is an example of a foot injury:

> My foot was on fire with pain as I could see the area around it turning red and blood oozing out. I felt so frustrated and stupid. . . . I felt tears forming

> in my eyes from my feelings of hopelessness and the throbbing pain in my foot. Trying to be brave, I walked/limped back to the restaurant expecting to see my boyfriend laughing at me because he saw what happened. . . . With each step I took to our table, the pain grew. I tried to act as if everything was fine so no one would pay attention to me. I wanted nothing more than to clean my wound so it wouldn't get infected and be told everything was going to be all right.

The genre of this description was romantic in its emphasis on the intensity of feelings directed to the foot and the boyfriend. She wanted consoling and care, and she wanted to be brave. Her pride was as injured as her foot.

The second example shared with the first the romantic genre:

> My boyfriend broke up with me. . . . I still love him. He loves me. He wants to get back together with me but not until he gets over some confusion he is going through. He wants to date other people. I want to die and I feel weak. I throw up all the time and cannot concentrate. I can't sleep and I have not eaten in three days 'cause I am not hungry.

In this hyperbolic passage, pain was a passion, a sickness. This pain of desire blocked other needs, such as hunger, sleep, and concentration. Her affliction demanded action, but she found no outlet save suffering and rejecting the loss by vomiting.

While this pain was passionate passivity, it was reflectively and actively passive. Pain inescapably entailed self-awareness: "During pain, around others, I feel hopeless, like a man stepping out of his body and watching it from the outside. . . . In fact, it seems as if the entire mind is concentrated on each moment equally, not being distracted." Was this an awareness of the self in pain or a painful self-awareness? Pain becomes now object, now subject. Bourke (2014) objects to the "ontologizing" of pain as an "it," but such objectification is part of the ambiguity of pain, which defies the neat distinctions of subject–object, dualism–monism, and body–mind.

The isolated landscape of pain

The being in the world of pain was one of fissures and distances. From a narrative of physical pain: "I became aware not only of the pain, but the fact that I was alone. I remember the mid-summer heat, the hot breeze, the feel of the rocks and dirt under me." Similarly, in a narrative of psychological pain: "The pain I felt was one of sorrow," wrote a young man with a speech impediment. "I felt so different . . . that I felt like curling up and letting the pain just run my life. It felt like when I would talk people would look at me like an outsider or a freak." This isolation led in many of the narratives either to a call for help or a response from someone coming to offer help. If pain constituted a break between the individual and the world, aid attempted to restore the person to ordinary life. This result finds support in Wall's (1979) conception of pain as a "need state." Along these lines, Esposito (2014) describes the manifestation of one's pain to others as an appeal, as a healing move, an effort to overcome isolation.

Differences between psychological and physical pain

The narratives portrayed physical and psychological pain as different types of pains. What were the differences?

Corporeal intrusion

Physical pain differed from psychological pain when the pain did not correspond to the interpersonal dynamics of the situation. Menstrual cramps felt "like my stomach was being clamped by a vice. . . . It sucked to feel so bad physically on what was supposed to be such a special Christmas." This woman had been anticipating joy, and the cramping intruded unbidden and thwarted enjoyment. Another woman made a similar contrast: "First there was the physical pain of cramps. Secondly, there was the mental anguish of not knowing what was wrong." Mental anguish was painful but of a different kind than the cramps. The cramps were a sheer presence, unavoidable and persistent, whereas the anguish concerned their significance. Some narratives saw the two types of pain supplementing each other:

> In dealing with "emotional pain," there is always physical pain that accompanies it. . . . At first, before I accepted the knowledge of her death, I had an uneasy feeling in my stomach, and the idea that I was dreaming.

The feeling in his stomach and the feeling of unreality differentiated physical and psychological pain that, nevertheless, occurred together.

Metaphoric substitution

Another narrator substituted a physical pain for a psychological pain: "I suffered from depression and turned to self-mutilation as a way, I think, to not concentrate on the mental pain, as well as remind myself that it could be worse." Self-mutilation shifted attention from a worse pain. This passage related physical and psychological pains metaphorically. They are alike in that both hurt; they differed in the location and the depth of the wounds. Nasio (2004), from a psychoanalytic perspective, shows the complexity of desires running through psychological and physical pain, with one substituting for the other.

Intimacy and social isolation

One narrator described feeling helpless in the face of psychological pain because it originated in desire: "No one would understand what you are going through so you don't want them to see your pain. After all, it's not physical and most likely cannot be helped by anything but time." The cultural construction of her pain as "not physical" implied that no remedy could cure it. Pain isolated her – "no one would understand" – and she flinched from rejection. Only by not thinking about her loss did she think that the pain would subside, even though this avoidance was central to the pain itself. Since this pain was not physical, if she could succeed in not thinking and not talking about it, it might not be there. Because it was not physical, she wished it to be not real.

Location and cause of wound

The narratives classified pain as either physical or psychological on the basis of the part of the self affected. Wounds visible to others are physical; those that are not might have been emotional – the dilemma that troubles people with chronic pain. Some causes were physical and others psychological, giving their character to the resulting pain. That some parts of the self and some causes were so defined indicates that we are dealing with meanings sedimented in common sense.

The two pains were most clearly differentiated in the narratives by their immediate antecedents. Getting hit by another football player differs from getting hit with a "good-bye" from a romantic partner. This distinction was not the same as that of severity or permanence, nor was it a difference between corporeal involvement or not (as a slap in the face would demonstrate). In this group of stories, every narrative of psychological pain began with the end of a relationship. In none of the physical pain narratives was that the case. The physical pain stories typically began with a fall or an accident. The difference had to do with the extent to which the narrator was the equivalent of a thing in the sequence of events that led to the pain. If one were functionally a thing in the situation, then the pain was physical. If one were a Thou, then the pain was emotional or psychological. This difference can easily be overstated, as the interpersonal realm is often a series of I–it relationships.

Consequences

Different activities followed from different kinds of pain. The performance of physical pain included medical care, taking that term in its broadest sense. With psychological pains, medical care occurred when there was a physical component, such as menstrual difficulties or a speech impediment. One narrator, after the end of a romantic relationship, underwent psychiatric treatment for depression. This is not, of course, to say that psychological pain does not wend its way to the physician's office (Martin & Brantley, 2004).

Pain as cultural performance

Pain is a performance of affliction, and as afflictions vary, so do the narratives. In the cultural milieu of these narrators, there are physical and psychological pains.

Despite the differences, one can substitute for the other, be described in terms of the other, be felt like the other, disable like the other. Pain is a performance by a person in a social situation. The results developed in this chapter support the idea, developed in earlier chapters, that pain is a cultural construction.

Similarity implies difference. As we have seen, psychological and physical pains are similar: We have found no phenomenological basis to reject classifying psychological pains as pains. Moreover, given the accounts of these pains as performances of affliction, they ought to be recognized as pain (see Biro, 2014, for a similar argument). There are many different kinds of pain – that of hunger, a burn, a broken leg, a chronic backache. Wounded pride and broken hearts also hurt.

Affliction, identity, suffering

Psychological pain is pain. If pain is a performance of affliction, then the assertion that psychological pain is pain is unproblematic. It becomes problematic only if biomedical criteria provide the defining characteristics of pain. Even the standard definitions of pain do not claim that biomedical indicators provide either the necessary or sufficient conditions of pain. If, however, we begin with the phenomenological concept of performance (considered further in the following chapter), then psychological pain as pain has a theoretical as well as an empirical grounding. Nevertheless, the addition of psychological pain as a kind of pain – and not as "pain" – continues the dualistic conception of pain that we noted previously: distinctions between pain as a sensation and emotional displeasure, for example. The distinctions between psychological and physical pains in the narratives drew upon sedimented cultural categories, such that pains in the chest following the loss of a loved one were psychological because the narrator did not consider them as needing a cardiologist's care. Embedded in the narrative classifications were references to dominant social institutions, such as medicine, which carve the person into psyche and soma. If we categorize the pains descriptively, however, what we find are various kinds of afflictions, neutral from the perspective of pain as performance to the distinction between the psychological and the physical. There are, for example, afflictions of loss of love, afflictions of menstruation, afflictions from wounds to feet and pride, and so on. Such a means of comprehending pain makes sense, however, if narrative and related performances ground conceptions of pain and not biomedicine.

In everyday accounts, subjects themselves define what is painful and define themselves in terms of how they reckon with pain, a point made in recent studies of pain narratives, which show that insofar as pain calls one's existence into question, the narratives are identity formative (Bauer, McAdams, & Pals, 2008; Eccleston, Williams, & Stainton Rogers, 1997; Jackson, 1994). Several of the narrators spoke of bravery in the face of pain. In other accounts, the pain of lost love served to define the self as one in love. Vernacular accounts position the subject as an active agent in defining himself or herself in performing pain. The "I" in affliction engages in self-formation in a variety of ways: with tears; with solitude;

with stories; with cries for help; with seeking medical aid; with lamenting loss, disability, and vulnerability. "I" am brave, hurt, weak, lost, dying, angry, or in pain: not as additions to a presupposed bare sensation, but as the performance of pain itself. Essential to pain, according to these narratives, is self-awareness. To be in pain is to say, in one way or another, "I" hurt and "it" hurts "me." There is ambiguity over whether pain concerns the "I" or the "it"; whether it is passivity or an activity; and whether it is, to employ the cultural categories, psychological or physical.

Critical reflections

The danger with recognizing psychological pain as pain is further medicalization. The thrust of this chapter has been to shift our thinking about pain more decisively from the anatomical image of the body to the lived body. If one begins with the body as lived, as felt by the person, then the bodily aspects of psychological pain are assured – that pain, like all pain, strikes the flesh. Acknowledgment of psychological pain as pain more clearly locates pain in the social world, a point made also by Biro (2014) and by MacDonald and Leary (2005). Pain has its structure in an embodied and social performance of a person. The further articulation of this as-yet imprecise formulation lies ahead in the next chapter. Here, we can conclude with the observation that everyday pain, no matter which type, can affect, disrupt, or at least trouble an entire existence. It is fundamentally an ethical performance.

Note

1 The research reported here first appeared in my 2000 article, "Pain in the Vernacular: Psychological and Physical," *Journal of Health Psychology, 5*, 305–314.

References

Bauer, J. J., McAdams, D. P., & Pals, J. L. (2008). Narrative identity and eudaimonic well-being. *Journal of Happiness Studies, 9*, 81–104. http://dx.doi.org/10.1007/s10902-006-9021-6

Biro, D. (2014). Psychological pain: Metaphor or reality. In R. Boddice (Ed.), *Pain and emotion in history* (pp. 53–65). New York, NY: Palgrave Macmillan.

Bourke, J. (2014). *The story of pain: From prayer to painkillers*. Oxford, England: Oxford University Press. http://dx.doi.org/10.14296/RiH/2014/1656

Eccleston, C. (2013). A normal psychology of everyday pain. *International Journal of Clinical Practice, 67*(Suppl. 178), 47–50.

Eccleston, C., & Crombez, G. (1999). Pain demands attention: A cognitive–affective model of the interruptive function of pain. *Psychological Bulletin, 125*, 356–366.

Eccleston, C., Williams, A. C., & Stainton Rogers, W. (1997). Patients' and professionals' understandings of the causes of chronic pain: Blame, responsibility and identity protection. *Social Science & Medicine, 45*, 699–709.

Esposito, J. (2014). Pain is a social construction until it hurts: Living theory on my body. *Qualitative Inquiry, 20*, 1179–1190.

Foucault, M. (1973). *The birth of the clinic* (A.M.S. Smith, Trans.). New York, NY: Vintage Books.

Gendlin, E. (1978–1979). *Befindlichkeit*: Heidegger and the philosophy of psychology. *Review of Existential Psychology and Psychiatry, 10*, 43–71.

Gündel, H., & Tölle, T. R. (2005). How physical pain may interact with psychological pain: Evidence for a mutual neurobiological basis of emotions and pain. In D. B. Carr, J. D. Loeser, & D. B. Morris (Eds.), *Narrative, pain and suffering* (pp. 87–112). Seattle, WA: IASP Press.

Jackson, J. E. (1994). Chronic pain and the tension between the body as subject and object. In T. J. Csordas (Ed.), *Embodiment and experience: The existential ground of culture and self* (pp. 201–228). Cambridge, England: Cambridge University Press.

Jackson, J. E. (2011). Pain and bodies. In F. E. Mascia-Lees (Ed.), *A companion to the anthropology of the body and embodiment* (pp. 370–387). Malden, MA: Wiley-Blackwell.

Leder, D. (1990). *The absent body*. Chicago, IL: University of Chicago Press.

MacDonald, G., & Leary, M. R. (2005). Why does social exclusion hurt? The relationship between social and physical pain. *Psychological Bulletin, 131*, 202–223. http://dx.doi.org/10.1037/0033-2909.131.2.202

Martin, P. D., & Brantley, P. J. (2004). Stress, coping, and social support in health and behavior. In J. M. Raczynsky & L. C. Leviton (Eds.), *Handbook of clinical health psychology* (Vol. 2, pp. 233–267). Washington, DC: American Psychological Association.

Masson, M., & Muirheid-Delacroix, B. (2014). La douleur morale: Historique et devinir d'un concept clinique. *Annales Médico-Psychologique, 172*, 139–145. http://dx.doi.org/10.1016/j.amp.2014.01.006

Mee, S., Bunney, B. G., Reist, C., Potkin, S. G., & Bunney, W. E. (2006). Psychological pain: A review of the evidence. *Journal of Psychiatric Research, 40*, 680–690. http://dx.doi.org/10.1016/j.psychires.2006.03.003

Merleau-Ponty, M. (1962). *Phenomenology of perception* (C. Smith, Trans.). New York, NY: Humanities Press.

Merleau-Ponty, M. (1969). Phenomenology and psychoanalysis: Preface to Hesnard's *Oeuvre de Freud*. In A. Fisher (Ed.), *The essential writings of Merleau-Ponty* (pp. 81–87). New York, NY: Harcourt, Brace & World.

Nasio, J.-D. (2004). *The book of love and pain: Thinking at the limit with Freud and Lacan* (D. Pettigrew & F. Raffoul, Trans.). Albany, NY: SUNY Press.

Staats, P. S., Hekmat, H., & Staats, A. W. (1996). The psychological behaviorism theory of pain: A basis for unity. *Pain Forum, 5*(3), 194–207.

Szasz, T. (1975). *Pain and pleasure: A study of bodily feelings* (2nd ed.). New York, NY: Basic Books. (Original work published 1957)

Wall, P. D. (1979). On the relation of injury to pain. *Pain, 6*, 253–264.

6

PHENOMENOLOGIES OF PAIN[1]

In this chapter, we will consider phenomenologies of pain. How has phenomenological thought contributed to answering the question *What is pain?* In the end, we will address pain as something that afflicts existence on multiple levels, at times simultaneously.

What is pain? How is pain?

So far, in studying some of the history of pain, the experience of chronic pain, and the experience of psychological pain, we have seen that pain confounds our dichotomies, asserting and contradicting them simultaneously: Pain is an *it*, pain is *I*; pain isolates me from the social world, pain exposes me, leaves me throbbing with every insult and look of scorn. This exposure can occur in differing ways: in the prepersonal lived body, through a wound or an illness; at the interpersonal level, felt bodily to be sure, of loss and grief; at the level of what is just and fair. This I/it is like an other whom I cannot face, afflicting me prior to any decision regarding it, belonging to a domain that in Hesiod's *Theogony* descends from Night and Strife, in a family that includes Fate, Doom, Death, Sleep, Old Age, Forgetfulness, and Starvation. How do we comprehend this child of Night and Strife?

Before reviewing major phenomenological contributions to the study of pain, I will briefly state the central finding. Phenomenologically speaking, we can understand pain in terms of "attunement." As an attunement, pain is a way people find themselves in the world. Pain is a "way-of-being" (Bourke, 2014, p. 8), a performance, an event. When we hurt, pain is *how* we are in the world. Like emotions, pain appraises what is happening. "If pain is not aversive," writes Sullivan (1996), "if it does not include a clearly negative affect, it is not recognizable as pain" (p. 208). Pain attunes a person toward action and in this way again is an emotional phenomenon. Moreover, pain as attunement has a cognitive aspect: In pain, the world is revealed in specific ways.

The phenomenological psychiatrist Medard Boss (1979) linked pain with sorrow as an attunement that reveals the gaps and fissures in the world. While in this chapter we will qualify this depiction, it contains an insight. In pain, one faces the fragmentary, frustrating, and incomplete character of existence. Hence, in the love of suffering – "philopassionism" (Cohen, 1995) – pain is embraced as a way of furthering this fragmentation because ordinary, mundane life separates us from the Divine. And in Greek or Shakespearean tragedy, the action of the drama shows someone undergoing the suffering of pain – not transcending it necessarily, but of necessity undergoing it. Pain is an undergoing that reveals something of human existence. A phenomenology of pain suggests that pain, in its being something we undergo, typically involuntarily, is nevertheless an opening onto the world – that is, an action that reveals something, even if that "something" is, in the extreme, disorder and destruction.

The lived body as the place of pain

Pain draws attention to the lived body, whether that pain is that of heartbreak or a heart attack. As much pain is medicalized, embodiment is experienced under the symbolic form of the anatomical image. Holloway, Sofaer-Bennett, and Walker (2007) observed that "those seeking help from pain clinics have a strong belief in organic pathology and demand biomechanical explanations" (p. 1458). In part, this results from entering a medical milieu; it also is a way to counter the "moral stigma" associated with a "lack of congruity between pain behaviours and objective medical findings" (p. 1458). This biomedical bias and the concomitant search for physical explanations turn attention away from the phenomenon of painful embodiment and toward a hidden source of the phenomenon – that is, the search for a biomedical cause invites psychosomatic dualism. Such a search may be appropriate, even if it means a flight from the phenomenon. "Cartesian dualism" is sometimes useful in dealing with pain (Gillies et al., 2004). Severe pain can reveal the lived body as not-me (Osborn & Smith, 2006) or not the real me (Edwards, Jones, Thacker, & Swisher, 2014). This ambiguity of the body as me and not-me is important to a phenomenology of pain.

Pain as sensory feeling

Perhaps the earliest extended phenomenology of pain, originally published in 1916, was Max Scheler's (1973) analysis of feelings and of values as their intentional objects. Scheler examined feelings in terms of their relatedness to the center of the life of the person and their relatedness to objects (Smith, 1978). Pain is a "sensible feeling" paired with pleasure. Sensible feelings have little connection to the center of personal life. Because pain occurs at the periphery of personal life, it is subordinate to emotions more central to personal existence. One can be in pain yet joy filled after having won a race, given birth to a child, or survived complex surgery. Sensible feelings are "states." A state is a condition of the person – how he or she is at this moment. Sensible feeling states are "extended and localized in specific parts of the lived body" (Scheler, 1973, p. 333) – that is, felt somewhere, unlike the deeper feelings, which are coextensive with the self. Sensible feelings can become the intentional objects of other acts (hence, one can suffer pain), but they themselves have no such object, their relationship with the objects that cause them being mediate (p. 256). Moreover, they exist only in actuality: I cannot "re-feel" them, as I can with deeper feelings, such as grief or love: As states, they are only *here* and they are only *now* – i.e., sensible feelings are conditions of the lived body.

For Scheler (1973), pain is a feeling state of the lived body, not of the objectified body. Pain, like other lived-body phenomena, has what Scheler called "extensionality," by which he meant that it can have a "side by side" and "sequential" character: Pain may alternate with an itch or be next to one, but it has no "fixed order" (p. 414) in objective space-time. Pain " 'spreads' 'across the back' or changes its place" (p. 413), but

> such lived-body phenomena are by no means "in" space, neither in an objective space (e.g., in an arm as an anatomic object) nor even in a phenomenal space. On the contrary, they share "non-spatiality" with everything belonging to the purely psychic
>
> *(p. 413)*

like thoughts and wishes. Here, Scheler asserted pain's mental nature.

Scheler described the relationships that sensible feelings have with "attributional objects" and with "causal objects." For example, if my hand hurts because I cut myself with a knife, the hand is the attributional object of that pain – it is where I feel it – and the knife is the causal object. For Scheler, pain's link with the causal object is indirect, whereas the link with the attributional object is direct: I feel the pain in my hand even if I do not know what cut me (Smith, 1978). Thus, for Scheler, pain has no intentional object; it is not "about" anything in the world. It is about the state of the person.

Because sensible feelings occur at a distance from the center of the self, they are subject to deliberate manipulation. Scheler (1973) observed that "*the more* feelings approach the level of *sensible* feeling-states, *the more* having or not having feelings is subject to *willing* and *not willing* (and consequently to practical methods of control)" (p. 336; italics in the original). This distance implies that "in principle, every kind of pain is subject to treatment by narcotics" (p. 336). Deeper feelings, including "purely psychic feelings" such as sadness and "spiritual feelings" such as bliss and despair, and, finally, love and hate are acts of the person, not states. They do not exist at an objective distance from one's self and so mean "me" in a way that sensible feelings do not.

Scheler's analysis in many ways harkens back to the early days of experimental psychology. The type of pain addressed conforms to some types of pain, especially acute pains, including those experimentally induced. This analysis does not grasp chronic pains, nor does it adequately address psychological pain as pain. It is valuable, however, in that Scheler raised the issue of pain as having variable relations with central aspects of life, a point important for psychological and moral pains.

Pain as performance

Drawing on physiological, biological, psychological, and philosophical analyses, the phenomenological physiologist F.J.J. Buytendijk (1962) concluded that functionality cannot explain pain. "Pain always comes too late" to serve as a signal of injury (pp. 95–96); it is "a given state of awareness of having been injured" (p. 100). He argued that the condition of possibility of pain "is to be sought for in animal existence itself" (p. 104) – namely, in that an animal has a point of view on its environment and can "place itself face to face with objects and its own body" (p. 104). Pain is *meaningful* as affliction, even if it is often *useless* functionally. Pain signifies "being afflicted"; it means "helplessness and perplexity" (p. 83).

Human pain further elaborates this basic sense of affliction because of human "eccentric positionality," a distance from self expressed in self-awareness and openness to possibility as possibility. A human being

> bears pain as something opposed to himself. Pain, which he senses directly, he also endures like any other animal, indirectly in its relationship to *himself*. Such pain lies outside the boundaries of the "vital" sphere: it is human in the primary sense of the word.
>
> *(Buytendijk, 1962, p. 87; italics in the original)*

In pain, the person undergoes affliction and "the more violent a pain, the deeper it penetrates, affecting not merely the 'body-self,' but our actual personality as well" (p. 114). Human eccentricity underlies what we have seen as the intractable dualism in the experience of pain. It is not specifically Cartesian, to be sure; it means viewing our bodies from a cognitive and emotional distance. Buytendijk's thesis is that pain "is characterized by an ambiguous relationship between the subject and its body. . . . We *are* in a certain way *our* body and we have a body" (p. 171; italics in the original).

Because pain signifies affliction, and because the vital (bodily) sphere does not exhaust human existence, Buytendijk (1962) examined aesthetic and ethical wounds as well as vital or biological wounds. When something is wrong or when something violates an aesthetic or moral order, one can suffer pain, and this not by analogy to physical pains. Quite the contrary, "*the 'vital' should be regarded as a particular manifestation of an ethical order rather than as a specific instance of conformity to the laws governing the 'vital' sphere*" (p. 137; italics in the original). Pain signifies destruction to the lived unity of an aspect of one's living, and our living is not confined to the vital sphere, as functionalism would claim.

Buytendijk (1962) thus rejected the thesis that pain is a sensation. He did differentiate between "sensory pain" and the feeling of pain, however, with the former being acute, localized bodily, and having an intentional object, making present, for example, the sharpness of an object. Such pain is sensory, because like touch, it reveals particular aspects of the immediately sensed world. On the other hand, "the feeling of pain" is not a phenomenon characterized by an intentional relationship. In feeling pain, a person "no longer experiences something confronting him, but *in* himself" (p. 125; italics in the original). Buytendijk found Scheler's notion that pain is a "sensory feeling" inadequate, for although it does account for acute, minor pains, it does not account for the ways that chronic and violent pains affect the deeply personal aspects of existence. Nor did Scheler address "the *dynamic* factor in pain" (p. 114; italics in the original). Pain is dynamic; it involves movement as well as feeling. Buytendijk emphasized the sensorimotor character of pain. Pain, Buytendijk wrote, is a "*performance* of the organism" (p. 115; italics in the original).

A performance is an act with gestural significance – that is, significance for others as well as for self. It is something a person does and, in so doing, it contributes to the making of the personal and social world in which the person dwells. A performance, then, is a construction of meaning. Pain is a particular type of performance. Pain is "*powerless* effort" (Buytendijk, 1962, p. 118; italics in the original). Pain is inability to act:

> To the inclination towards flight which follows a painful stimulus is added the *inability* to escape from pain. This, then, is the peculiar character of pain: to burn, gnaw, and oppress the body in various ways so that its adequate expression is a scream, in fact "an ineffective effort."
>
> *(p. 121; italics in the original)*

One cannot flee it. Buytendijk concluded that the essence of pain is "to disrupt man's inner 'vital' and psychic structure with incomparable force, but without attacking his personal existence" (p. 132). The literature on biographical disruption, especially with chronic pain, would dispute this claim of Buytendijk's. Thus, his last phrase is not quite right, because pain does attack personal existence, but insofar as we suffer, personal existence remains. What Buytendijk meant is that pain, because it is something that one enacts and constructs, has the possibility of being elaborated in the innumerable ways of culture. One can attempt to flee it by seeking remedies, distraction, inebriation, sleep, and death. One can suffer it bravely or pursue it with spiritual fervor. The bitter truth is that while pain confronts the individual, it also is internal to the person's existence (p. 125). Pain cannot be removed the way a thorn causing pain can be removed.

This notion of pain as performance receives support from recent phenomenological work: "Pain turns out to be 'a blocked movement of flight' . . . it cannot be ignored, disconnected, deactivated, nor can it be accepted or integrated, it can only be suffered" (Serrano de Haro, 2012, p. 231, quoting Grüny, 2004). Pain is a specific kind of performance, an active passivity. Pain shapes *how* the world and all within it, including the self, appear. Essential to pain is an aversion or repulsion on the part of the self (Buytendijk, 1962; Levinas, 1988). Even if pain is cultivated, the painful is something to be repulsed. In pain, there occurs a backward movement of subjectivity which, although ineffective, continues as long as pain endures. Pain infects subjectivity, being a state that is an act, a passive performance. We saw this combination of passivity and activity in chronic pain, where the world becomes a prison, where one finds oneself homeless, with no place to be. The performance of pain is both a passivity and a performance.

Finally, following one connotation of the word *performance*, we can affirm Moscoso's (2012) assertion that "pain is a drama" (p. 6). This drama for Moscoso has a precise form, one in keeping with phenomenological observations: "It displays a dynamic structure that includes a moment of rupture that demands reparation" (p. 6). The sometimes illusory plot of this drama is that pain should cease. Bourke's (2014) detailed accounts of historical possibilities for the performance of pain – people "do" pain in her terms – indicate that the performance of pain takes place in specific social and historical milieus. Finally, as performance, pain is a display, for others and for self. The privacy of pain is social.

The lived body as the place of pain

Jean-Paul Sartre (1956) took up Scheler's distinction between sensible feelings and intentional feelings, calling the former ways "in which consciousness *exists* its contingency" (p. 331; italics in the original), distinguishing between a prereflective and a reflective grasp of pain, differentiating levels of constitution of reflective meaning. Prereflectively, pain (in the eyes, in his example) "is totally void of intentionality . . . pain is *precisely the eyes* in so far as consciousness 'exists them' " (p. 332; italics in the original). Pain is *here* and *now* as "consciousness, its *being-there*, its attachment to the world, in short the peculiar contingency of the act of reading" (p. 333; italics in the original). This "pain consciousness" is the way I am at this moment, the way I am "inserted" into the world. At this moment, I have no cognitive or emotional distance from pain. Like Buytendijk, Sartre pointed to a backward move of consciousness in pain, "a wrenching away from self. . . . Pain-consciousness is a project toward a further consciousness which would be empty of all pain" (p. 333). Sartre observed that "the inexpressible which one wishes to flee is rediscovered at the heart of this wrenching away" (p. 333) – pain is ineffective, helpless flight.

In a first reflective grasp, we find that each pain has a temporality and rhythm: "It is given as a living thing which has its form, its own duration, its habits" (Sartre, 1956, p. 336). This quasi-subject is not a true other. It is almost outside consciousness, but (using common imagery) "it fastens on to consciousness with all its teeth, penetrates consciousness with all its notes; and *these teeth, these notes are my consciousness*" (p. 337; italics in the original). Pain in this first reflection is an

> affective object. One directs oneself first toward one's pain so as to hate it, to endure it with patience, to apprehend it as unbearable, sometimes to love it, to rejoice in it (if it foretells a release, a cure), to evaluate it in some way.
>
> *(p. 337)*

This quasi-subject is the object of an emotional consciousness.

The two moments Sartre described – lived pain and object pain – to use Toombs's terms (1992, p. 31), coexist all the more insistently the more intense the pain is. The first moment, lived pain, has no intentional relationship with objects. It is not yet an "it"; instead, it is me, what I am at this moment. It resembles other "states" of the lived body that I am prereflectively. This possibility shows the limitation of Scheler's hierarchy: Intense pain consumes the person as deeply as love, rage, fear, anxiety, and hate. Object pain manifests the injury, the division within the self, a breakdown, which Bakan (1968) called "telic decentration." In pain, I not only objectify part of me, I can consent to its being carved away with a knife. Before 1846, when ether was introduced into surgery, in the anguish of deciding to submit to the steel, people inescapably faced contradictions of being and having a body that pain imposes, as we have seen. The duality of being and having seems insurmountable – that is a meaning of pain.

Later phenomenological contributions on pain also focus on the lived body. In so doing, they move decisively away from the anatomical image of the body to embodiment. Leder (1984–1985, 1990, 1992) examined pain as a sensation in light of Merleau-Ponty's (1962) critique of the psychology of sensation. Understood phenomenologically, sensations are ways of being present to the world. Pain offers only contradictions, for while it provides "a mode of communication between the self and its physical and social surroundings" (Leder, 1984–1985, p. 261), pain is not a moment of self-transcendence but "the latent possibility of the sensory world to trap us in the present" (p. 256). In pain, the self is pinned down in place, in an "unmaking" of the world (Scarry, 1985), but "pain's inward pull simultaneously thrusts us away" (Leder, 1984–1985, p. 257) from the here and the now and the flesh, a consequence of the repulsion that constitutes pain. Even as pain is an evil, so also it has at times a "positive role" – for example, in "the accompaniment of birth, not only of babies, but of physical and emotional achievements" (Leder, 1984–1985, p. 259), although the evaluation of pain as good or bad here depends upon something like Scheler's hierarchy of values. Pain can at once demonstrate that we are flesh and simultaneously that the body is alien, uncannily other, not-me, that the body is a tomb.

Olivier's (2007) recent phenomenology of pain concluded that "pain is always bodily pain: I am a perceiving body and as a perceiving body I am in pain" (p. 48). He thereby furthered the critique of the sensation theory, arguing that sensing is not prior to cognition but a manner of knowing, and he advanced a critique of the theory that pain consists of two components, sensations and emotions: "Sensations, emotions and cognitions are . . . modes of perception, that is, ways in which I qua body relate to others and myself" (p. 38). Whatever I do is a sensorimotor act of me as lived body, and sensing, emoting, and thinking are abstractions of such acts. Olivier further specified pain as perception "*bound to hurt, affliction, or agony*" (p. 51; italics in the original), thereby indicating modalities in the ways that pain "disturbs" existence in both "physical" and "psychological" ways.

The field of pain

Phenomenologically, then, pain is a sensorimotor performance. Along these lines, Schrag (1982) deconstructed the dichotomy of subjective and objective that has served to conceptualize pain. This dichotomy is rooted in the metaphor of inside/outside, which "provides a grid for sorting out that which is internally experienced by the subject in pain from the externally observable, overt, bodily behavior" (p. 109). We have seen instances of this metaphor repeatedly – for example, in Merskey and Spear's distinction between pain as subjective experience and the causes of pain and in Fordyce's focus on pain behavior in contrast to pain experience. However, the metaphor fails for pain, because pain cannot simply be called an experience; it is also activity. The behaviorist ignoring of pain experience, while promising from one perspective, fails because "pain behavior" tacitly refers to inner experience (p. 112). Schrag proposed a new metaphor of "'configurative behavior' to bind together a number of allied features which characterize the phenomenon of being in pain" (pp. 113–114). These features are "(1) the field of presentative phases of consciousness; (2) the field of embodiment; (3) the field of attitudinal posture and praxis; and (4) the field of existential temporality" (p. 114). Schrag wrote that all aspects of the conscious field form and inform pain: "Sensation, emotion, memory, imagination, and even conception conspire in different ways to structure the phenomenon of pain" (p. 115). Pain configures the field of consciousness as such. Schrag addressed the active–passive dichotomy, asserting that the intentionality of consciousness must be understood in "a wider context . . . in which the specifications of a passive and an active role are relatively late arrivals" (p. 116). This is important for pain, since sensation and feeling are generally seen as passive acts, thoughts and judgments as active ones, and pain spans them both. Pain is a passivity in that typically it happens without regard to personal acts; it is an activity in many ways, especially in the ways it is taken up and lived.

As a passive activity, pain is a *how* of one's existing, one's *noesis*, to use the Husserlian term (Idhe, 2012). Every *how* correlates with a *what* or *noema*, and the *noema* is the field – spatial, temporal, social – of the phenomenon. Our view of the field broadening, "pain is a mode of existing in the world against a background of attitudes to be assumed, projects to be undertaken, tasks to be performed, and goals to be realized" (Schrag, 1982, p. 120). Pain integrates itself into my tasks, my social relations, and my situation. Finally, the field of pain has its temporality, and Schrag, with Sartre, saw it intending a painless future. Pain has its eschatology. The temporality of pain, as one hopes and works for release, is not an objective temporality. In pain, time can virtually stop completely.

A central conclusion from the this review is that pain is something not done, ineffective or helpless action, failed repulsion: This dynamic helps specify pain as performance. The Heideggerian concept of "attunement" can further this understanding of pain, deepening and not resolving the paradoxes it presents.

Attunements

Feelings as attunements

According to Heidegger (1985), "being-in-the-world is . . . constantly being summoned by the *threatening* and *non-threatening* character of the world" (p. 254; italics in the original). We always find ourselves so summoned, and "this does not mean that the caring Dasein thus construes the world 'subjectively.' . . . Rather, the caring in-being discovers the world in its meaningfulness" (pp. 254–255). The general term for this self-finding and world discovery Heidegger called *Befindlichkeit* or "attunement." Gendlin (1978–1979) indicated that attunement provides a way to look anew at affective life, which has been relegated to the subjective realm. Heidegger's term, Gendlin suggested, could be translated as "how-are-you-ness" or as "self-finding," in order to capture the sense of "the reflexivity of finding oneself; feeling; and being situated" (p. 44). Attunements – including feelings, moods, dispositions, and emotions – provide limited openings to the world. An attunement "precedes and eliminates the distinction between *inside and outside*, as well as between *self and others*. Similarly, it alters [the] *affective/cognitive*" dichotomy (Gendlin, 1978–1979, p. 47; italics in the original). A metaphor may help: Pain is atmospheric, in that pain can permeate all one's self and world. One lives *in* pain.

Attunements have their own implicit understanding or grasp of what is going on, as "understanding is always attuned" (Heidegger, 1953/1996, p. 134). According to Gendlin, an understanding is felt bodily as an attunement. This "feeling" for things or "felt bodily sense" (Gendlin, 1978–1979) is revelatory of the world and not only of the self. Together with understanding, attunement has "its spoken articulation" (Gendlin, 1978–1979, p. 45), for understanding is not understanding if it does not fulfill itself in speech. "Speech" here need not mean literally words; rather, it means expression, and it can include gestural display. So even when a person cannot articulate pain verbally, pain gestures and behavior manifest how the person is attuned.

Pain as attunement

Medard Boss (1979) discussed pain in considering several attunements: love, hate, anger, serenity, anxiety, and sorrow. He addressed pain as a mode of sorrow. A sorrowful attunement occurs in an existence "when it experiences a break or rupture in its relationship to a close human acquaintance or some cherished object, but the object of sorrow is not lost with this rupture" (p. 113). In sorrow, one comes to grips with the "breaking, rending, and damaging of existential relationships" (p. 114). Like Buytendijk, Boss reversed the usual way of thinking of the relationship of psychological and physical pain. Typically, psychologists view psychological pain as being based on physical pain (see Mee et al., 2006). For Boss, what we call physical pain is the attunement to a rupture that affects the "bodying forth" of existence: "Will sorrow – inner pain [–] be understood on the basis of bodily pain, or does bodily pain depend, rather, on sorrow, the recognition of a flaw running through the abundance of relational possibilities?" (Boss, p. 114). He referred to a case of a woman injured in an automobile accident: "In her pain there was no awareness of the automobile bumper that had splintered her leg. What the pain told her at first was only that her existence had been hit hard and injured" (p. 189). In pain, she lived a fractured existence with broken possibilities. Pain signified exposure and the contingency of life's possibilities.

For Boss (1979), "bodily pain always inheres in some injury done to a person's relatedness to the world – that is, to the person's very existing" (p. 212). Bodily pain is a narrow attunement, we might say, for it "heralds exclusively injury to our ability to body forth our relatedness to the world" (p. 212). Because of this narrow focus, sorrow is the existential ground of physical pain: "The psychic pain of sorrow reveals the fundamental, existential laceration of *Da-sein*; physical pain only permits us to perceive partial impairments in the bodily sphere of ways of being" (p. 212). Physical pain, according to Boss, is a sorrowful attunement. However, intense or chronic pain is not so narrow; its reach extends beyond "partial impairments," as it affects all of living. Pain as a modality of sorrow may account for the frequent association of chronic pain and depression (Banks & Kerns, 1996; Lima, Alves, & Turato, 2014). I say this with caution, since depression is not simply sorrow, even in Boss's existential terms.

Boss's insight becomes clearer if we substitute the obsolete English word *dolor* for *pain*. Meaning at once what Boss has been calling bodily pain and sorrow, *dolor* names an awareness of brokenness, injury, and loss that is neutral with respect to the terms *physical* and *mental*. Pain – dolor – discloses the flawed nature of existence.

Heidegger (1971) discussed pain as presented in a poem of Georg Trakl. Heidegger wrote:

> But what is pain? Pain rends. It is the rift. But it does not tear apart into dispersive fragments. Pain indeed tears asunder, it separates, yet so that at the same time it draws everything to itself, gathers it to itself. Its rending, as a separating that gathers, is at the same time that drawing which, like the pen-drawing of a plan or sketch, draws and joins together what is held apart in separation. Pain is the joining agent in the rending that divides and gathers. Pain is the joining of the rift. The joining is the threshold.
>
> *(p. 204)*

Here is a thinking that steps outside of the dichotomies of subjective/objective and useful/useless that have defined psychology's theories of pain. Caputo (1993) took up the metaphor that pain is a threshold in his critique of Heidegger:

> The body in pain clears the clearing in an originary way, opens up the space in which we dwell from the start, generates the lines of force that are inscribed in human space. . . . Pain opens up the distinction between what is

> essential and what is not, what matters and what does not. Pain is a threshold that opens up the divide of human space, but this is the kind of pain which cuts flesh or breaks hearts, which divides families or friends or lovers, the pain enforced by disease, separation, or death.
>
> *(pp. 167–168)*

This passage amplifies what we have seen about pain as attunement: In feeling pain, one occupies a threshold. We previously encountered this place of pain in examining chronic pain, where it appeared as a kind of no-place. The locus of this threshold is first of all the lived body, but moreover, and not only metaphorically, places of anguish, injury, disease, and violence.

Olivier (2007) objected, with reason, to characterizing all pain as rending. This metaphor accounts for some extreme pain, but what about the garden variety of aches and hurts that do not shake us to the core? As a more general term for the attunement of pain, Olivier suggested "disturbance." Some pains, whether of loss or injury, cut existence, but not to the quick. Rupture, in this reading, is a more serious disturbance. Pain shows itself as a performance at the thresholds of existence, where one is attuned to the disturbances and ruptures within oneself and the world.

Pain as a threshold

As a rupture or disturbance – a threshold, an attunement – pain forms a "from-where" of human presence, opening up the person to things that elude painless ways of being. Pain is an undergoing, an affliction, and an older term, *passion*, captures something of the undergoing that pain entails. The phenomenological psychologist Bernd Jager (1989) discerned the "strange affinity that pain, suffering, and passion hold for each other" (p. 220), a point amplified by Sipiora (2012), who called all attunements passions. Pain is a passion in that pain is a drive for deliverance. Severe pain potentially opens onto "the fateful and tragic dimensions of human life" (Jager, 1989, p. 220). Jackson (1994) found this transformation among chronic pain sufferers: "Just like the ineffable worlds of dreams, day-dreams, or deep religious or musical experience, the pain-full world has its own system of meaning" (pp. 213–214). To those not in pain, the person in pain can seem unreasonable and needy, just as are those in the throes of rage or erotic love. They have been transported out of the paramount reality of the everyday (Schutz, 1973) into an elsewhere, where the boundaries between types of passions blur.

Passion – following Jager's (1978) phenomenology of passion – involves a passage through a constraining point and promises release. Anger, eros, sleep, and death all have moments of crisis: the outburst, the orgasm, the fall into slumber, the dying. Before that moment, there is a building of tension; after it, release, peace, calm, stillness. That is the narrative of passion that Jager described. Pain, especially severe pain, resembles this account, but it is metaphorical to call all pain a passion, pure and simple. The passions find their release in an oblivion, whereas chronic pain can make oblivion impossible: hence the appeal of opiates. The passion becomes unbearable when the upwelling fails to hurl us across the gap into release. Pain thus resembles the passions in this, at least – that it too entails a crisis or threshold – but in pain, we stay at the threshold.

Pain is a peculiar existential threshold. A threshold is a passage between two states, and the particularity of pain is that it blocks passage. Intense pain is agony because it does not let us go. Edward Casey (1993) developed a phenomenology of place, showing how "body and place belong together" (p. 45). Being in the world is a "being-in-place" (p. 314). Pain's place, a threshold, defines the place of pain as a *here*: the body, the situation, the room I cannot leave, the love or the job that I have lost. The place of pain is a threshold with the crossing blocked. Lingering and escape are both impossible. Of pain we sometimes say *I cannot stand it*, meaning one cannot tolerate being *in* pain. Pain is a threshold phenomenon. Pain is a thwarted desire to cross the threshold to a promised release. One person with chronic pain described it in these terms:

> You've got to understand when you've got this kind of a pain you can't do nothing. You have to get up, get down, get up, get down. Because if you sit too long it feels like your whole hind end is just, it's hurting real bad, I mean your whole left hind end is hurting really bad to the point where you have to get up.

He found himself restless and irritable:

> At that time I was becoming irritable. I wasn't at the point of drinking, I wasn't at the point of taking a whole lot of medicine, but I was irritable. I was ready to cut somebody's head off if they tried to talk to me about something that was not right.

Those points came soon enough, and he drank, and he obtained painkillers illegally. Restlessness, explosions of anger, and inebriation are attempts to flee the agony of pain and regain the everyday world. Pain pins the person down, making existence coextensive with the spatiality of the body in pain. It is essential to pain to seek escape. Pain the place cannot be inhabited; like a threshold, there is a next step – if only it could be made.

Minor pains do not rise typically to the level of passion, just as not all anger is rage. Minor pains disturb existence, placing us at thresholds, marking "cuts" in living. Instead of trapping one at a threshold, they may simply make for a pause at one. Pain is a "primal separation" (Clark, 1977, p. 336) that splits and connects self and world.

The intentionality of pain

A number of phenomenological studies address the intentionality of pain, none better than Honkasalo's (2000). Describing the ways that two of her interviewees lived in pain, she wrote that they "created the intentional object of their pain by retaining a passionate relationship to *both of their worlds*, before and after the onset of pain" (p. 205; italics in the original). Pain opened a fissure, and these two people grieved something that they had loved and lost: "The feeling I got when listening to him [one of the participants] is a feeling of sadness after a love story" (p. 203). While nothing requires that loss be lived in precisely this way, it is one existential possibility, and a phenomenon is its possibilities (Idhe, 2012). Other phenomenological researchers have noticed something similar. Pain is the experience of loss:

> The major finding of the study is, therefore, the primacy of existential pain and suffering in the lives of many of the residents who participated in the study. There seemed to be an ongoing work of reconciliation and adjustments to different losses and existential changes which for many went well but some seemed to be stuck. The residents can all be placed on a continuum of an imaginary line – "the work of reconciliation to losses in life."
>
> *(Gudmannsdottir & Halldorsdottir, 2009, p. 321)*

Participants in this study varied as to the extent to which they were reconciled to loss, a point made by an earlier study (Murphy & Fischer, 1983), which describes the consequences of back injury on working men:

> When an able-bodied, hard-working man, who has always been and expects to continue to be active in this manner, undergoes back injury in a work accident, his entire way of life becomes vulnerable. The disruption of his prior relationships to others, himself and his world is concomitantly a threat that he may no longer be the person he was. As the opportunities of the past close off, he is confronted with choosing who he will be. He takes up the injury in terms of the most personally viable self and future which he finds available.
>
> *(p. 292)*

This sense of division in existence was found in a number of studies as reviewed by Osborn and Rodham (2010): "The participants gave extensive accounts of their distress and talked about how they struggled to maintain a stable, coherent or valued sense of either being a person or being treated like a person" (p. 5). Not that the rift is necessarily a "biographical disruption" (Bury, 1982), although it might be; it also might be a disturbance in a biography, perhaps as one gets older. That does not make it any less poignant: *Mais où sont les neiges d'antan? But where are the snows of yesteryear?* So asked the poet Villon about lost beauty. A recent article by Jennifer Esposito (2014), which included an autoethnography, describes a descent into loss and eventual transformation.

The very dynamism of pain bids us to consider its intentionality. Pain the threshold, the rift, the disturbance, the loss, is dolor. Its place incites cries to cross the threshold. Its temporality points beyond itself, all the more insistently the more it lingers. A fitting image of this deformation of the human condition is Hell – endless suffering. All writers on pain have found themselves addressing eschatology, because that is the dynamism of pain. Pain the threshold opens up radically different possibilities: Growing pains and mortal wounds are both pains, because of the duality, the duplicity of pain.

Critical reflections

Phenomenological considerations of pain show that pain cannot be simply understood as something bodily or as something mental. Like other phenomena, pain takes place. Its place we have described as a threshold. A threshold promises passage from one location to another, and the agony of pain – in pain behavior of writhing and restlessness – is that it can affix us to this threshold. Pain is a performance attuned to the thresholds of disturbances and ruptures, of loss and lack, of existence. This threshold is the "no place to be" of pain. Pain is a performance in this no-place. Pain is a drama enacted there, and these dramas include, as we have seen, the mental and the physical. These two are clearly differentiated, even as they have much in common, in large part because social institutions, especially medicine, enforce a difference.

So where does this account leave us? For one thing, pain is not simply an object of medicine or the natural sciences. It is a way of existing and, as such, it reveals the world in ways that nothing else does. It reveals the gaps, the fissures, the limits of existence. This phenomenology provides the raw material for understanding the ways in which individuals and societies construct pain in particular ways. The thresholds that pain reveals, moreover, occur in different aspects or dimensions of existence, from the "merely" physical to the emotional, aesthetic, and moral. Different ways of life will mark these boundaries in differing ways.

Pain is a stern teacher. There is, therefore, something we can call sacred about pain, in the sense that being in pain, a person attends and encounters the discord and groundlessness of our existence. Pain is not only a symbol of disorder; it is the very realization of it. Pain is a condition that calls for alleviation, and we all need support because of the gulf beneath our feet. In this condition, we foresee a painless future, a vision that may be illusory. However, pain is not simply something undergone: It is also something we enact. To that topic we now turn.

Note

1 Parts of this chapter were drawn from an earlier publication: Robert Kugelmann, "Pain, Place, Pathos" from *Challenges to Theoretical Psychology*, W. Maiers, B. Bayer, B. D. Esgalhado, R. Jorna, & E. Schraube (Eds.), Concord, ON, Canada: Captus Press, 1999, pp. 182–190. Reprinted with permission of Captus Press Inc.

References

Bakan, D. (1968). *Disease, pain and sacrifice: Toward a psychology of suffering*. Chicago, IL: University of Chicago Press.

Banks, S. M., & Kerns, R. D. (1996). Explaining high rates of depression in chronic pain: A diathesis-stress framework. *Psychological Bulletin, 119*(1), 95–110. http://dx.doi.org/10.1037/0033-2909.119.1.95

Boss, M. (1979). *Existential foundations of medicine and psychology* (S. Conway & A. Cleaves, Trans.). New York, NY: Aronson.

Bourke, J. (2014). *The story of pain: From prayer to painkillers.* Oxford, England: Oxford University Press. http://dx.doi.org/10.14296/RiH/2014/1656

Bury, M. (1982). Chronic illness as biographical disruption. *Sociology of Health and Illness, 4*, 167–182.

Buytendijk, F.J.J. (1962). *Pain: Its modes and functions* (E. O'Shiel, Trans.). Chicago, IL: University of Chicago Press.

Caputo, J. D. (1993). *Demythologizing Heidegger.* Bloomington: Indiana University Press.

Casey, E. S. (1993). *Getting back into place: Toward a renewed understanding of the place-world.* Bloomington: Indiana University Press.

Clark, O. (1977). Heidegger and the mystery of pain. *Man & World, 10*, 334–350.

Cohen, E. (1995). Towards a history of European physical sensibility: Pain in the later Middle Ages. Science in Context, 8, 47–74.

Edwards, I., Jones, M., Thacker, M., & Swisher, L. L. (2014). The moral experience of the patient with chronic pain: Bridging the gap between first and third person ethics. *Pain Medicine, 15*, 364–378.

Esposito, J. (2014). Pain is a social construction until it hurts: Living theory on my body. *Qualitative Inquiry, 20*, 1179–1190.

Gendlin, E. (1978–1979). *Befindlichkeit*: Heidegger and the philosophy of psychology. *Review of Existential Psychology and Psychiatry, 10*, 43–71.

Gillies, V., Harden, A., Johnson, K., Reavey, P., Strange, V., & Willig, C. (2004). Women's collective constructions of embodied practices through memory work: Cartesian dualism in memories of sweating and pain. *British Journal of Social Psychology, 43*, 99–112.

Grüny, C. (2004). *Zerstörte Erfahrung: Eine Phänomenologie des Schmerzes.* Würzburg, Germany: Königshausen & Neumann.

Gudmannsdottir, G. D., & Halldorsdottir, S. (2009). Primacy of existential pain and suffering in residents in chronic pain in nursing homes: A phenomenological study. *Scandanavian Journal of Caring Sciences, 23*, 317–327.

Heidegger, M. (1971). Language. In *Poetry, language, thought* (A. Hofstadter, Trans., pp. 187–210). New York, NY: Harper Colophon.

Heidegger, M. (1985). *History of the concept of time: Prolegomena* (T. Kisiel, Trans.). Bloomington: Indiana University Press.

Heidegger, M. (1996). *Being and time* (J. Stambaugh, Trans.). Albany, NY: SUNY Press. (Original work published 1953)

Holloway, I., Sofaer-Bennett, B., & Walker, J. (2007). The stigmatization of people with chronic back pain. *Disability and Rehabilitation, 29*, 1456–1464.

Honkasalo, M.-L. (2000). Chronic pain as a posture towards the world. *Scandinavian Journal of Psychology, 41*(3), 197–208.

Idhe, D. (2012). *Experimental phenomenology: Multistabilities* (2nd ed.). Albany, NY: SUNY Press.

Jackson, J. E. (1994). Chronic pain and the tension between the body as subject and object. In T. J. Csordas (Ed.), *Embodiment and experience: The existential ground of culture and self* (pp. 201–228). Cambridge, England: Cambridge University Press.

Jager, B. (1978). Toward a phenomenology of the passions. In R. S. Valle & M. King (Eds.), *Existential-phenomenological alternatives for psychology* (pp. 341–357). New York, NY: Oxford University Press.

Jager, B. (1989). Transformation of the passions: Psychoanalytical and phenomenological perspectives. In R. S. Valle & S. Halling (Eds.), *Existential-phenomenological perspectives in psychology*. New York, NY: Plenum Press, 217–231.

Leder, D. (1984–1985). Toward a phenomenology of pain. *Review of Existential Psychology and Psychiatry, 19*, 255–266.

Leder, D. (1990). *The absent body*. Chicago, IL: University of Chicago Press.

Leder, D. (1992). The experience of pain and its clinical implications. *Philosophy and Medicine, 40*, 95–105.

Levinas, E. (1988). Useless suffering. In R. Bernasconi & D. Wood (Eds.), *The provocation of Levinas: Rethinking the other* (pp. 156–167). New York, NY: Routledge.

Lima, D. D., Alves, V.L.P., & Turato, E. R. (2014). The phenomenological-existential comprehension of chronic pain: Going beyond the standing healthcare models. *Philosophy, Ethics, and Humanities in Medicine, 9*(2). http://dx.doi.org/10.1186/1747-5341-9-2

Mee, S., Bunney, B. G., Reist, C., Potkin, S. G., & Bunney, W. E. (2006). Psychological pain: A review of the evidence. *Journal of Psychiatric Research, 40*, 680–690. http://dx.doi.org/10.1016/j.psychires.2006.03.003

Merleau-Ponty, M. (1962). *Phenomenology of perception* (C. Smith, Trans.). New York, NY: Humanities Press.

Moscoso, J. (2012). *Pain: A cultural history* (S. Thomas & P. House, Trans.). New York, NY: Palgrave Macmillan.

Murphy, M. A., & Fischer, C. T. (1983). Styles of living with low back injury: The continuity dimension. *Social Science & Medicine, 17*, 291–297.

Olivier, A. (2007). *Being in pain*. Frankfurt, Germany: Lang.

Osborn, M., & Rodham, K. (2010). Insights into pain: A review of qualitative research. *Reviews in Pain, 4*(1), 2–7.

Osborn, M., & Smith, J. (2006). Living with a body separate from the self: The experience of the body in chronic benign low back pain: An interpretative phenomenological analysis. *Scandinavian Journal of Caring Sciences, 20*, 216–222.

Sartre, J.-P. (1956). *Being and nothingness* (H. Barnes, Trans.). New York, NY: Philosophical Library.

Scarry, E. (1985). *The body in pain: The making and unmaking of the world*. New York, NY: Oxford University Press.

Scheler, M. (1973). *Formalism in ethics and non-formal ethics of values* (M. S. Frings & R. L. Funk, Trans.). Evanston, IL: Northwestern University Press.

Schrag, C. (1982). Being in pain. In V. Kestenbaum (Ed.), *The humanity of the ill* (pp. 101–124). Knoxville: University of Tennessee Press.

Schutz, A. (1973). *Collected papers I: The problem of social reality* (4th ed.). The Hague, Netherlands: Nijhoff.

Serrano de Haro, A. (2012). New and old approaches to the phenomenology of pain. *Studia Phaenomenologica, 12*, 227–237.

Sipiora, M. (2012). Sorrow, existence, and the humanities. *The Humanistic Psychologist, 40*, 258–261. http://dx.doi.org/10.1080.08873267.2012.696506

Smith, Q. (1978). Max Scheler and the classification of feelings. *Journal of Phenomenological Psychology, 9*, 114–138.

Sullivan, M. D. (1996). Pain as emotion. *Pain Forum, 5*, 208–209.

Toombs, S. K. (1992). *The meaning of illness: A phenomenological account of the different perspectives of physician and patient*. Dordrecht, Netherlands: Kluwer Academic.

7

PAIN AS A SIGN[1]

Pain is an attunement to the flaws in existence, to disharmony and disorder. In an embodied sense, pain is a way of disclosing the world. In this chapter, I develop this idea, drawing on the semiotics of Charles Sanders Peirce. Peirce's theory of the sign allows for a variety of ways of knowing the world. As Merleau-Ponty said, there are many ways for consciousness to be consciousness, and explicitly discursive knowing is but one of them. Pain can be brutally inarticulate yet still revelatory.

Pain as a symptom and a sign

Consider pain as a medical symptom. When I am afflicted with pain, I confront my own mortality, often much too closely. Pain the symptom means *me*. Yet even as I feel it, it is caught like a bug on the flypaper of a socially constructed reality. In the instant that I feel pain, it already has social significance. It enters chains of discursive and other acts involving me with others and with institutions. I interpret it as meaning something – or meaning nothing. In short, pain as a symptom signifies.

The intersection of the personal and the consensually validated is a key concern of critical approaches to health. Studies of health beliefs and representations, expert and lay knowledge systems, discourse and power relationships in health systems, and the economics of healthcare delivery, to name but a few, turn on the pivot of the intersection of the individual and the social. In this chapter, we turn to the construction of our subjectivities and objectivities through pain as a way of knowing self and world. The semiotics of Charles Sanders Peirce advances the critical approach to pain that we have so far pursued. Semiotics (the study of signs) directs inquiry to precisely those moments, events, and places within human activity where meaning is constructed, enacted, and communicated. I shall explore

Peirce's semiotics by addressing complaints of pain in the medical context – that is, as a symptom. Even physical pain, as we shall see, grasps and reveals the world, and not only as a biomedical symptom. That insight will be a prelude to a study of moral pain in the concluding chapter.

Medical symptoms, medical signs, and felt bodily sense

In medical contexts, pain is, above all, a symptom, meaning something that the patient reports feeling or happening. Symptoms are *subjective*. A sign in medical terms, by contrast, is *objective*, something the physician detects. The difference between the two presupposes the dichotomies – subjective and objective, mental and physical, lay and expert – that a critical approach to health finds inadequate to account for health and illness. In Peirce's terms, both the medical symptom and the medical sign are types of signs because they both signify something to someone.

Now, a medical sign may not be felt: High blood pressure and cancerous moles may not produce medical symptoms, and their coconstitution as medically significant may require formal involvement in the medical system. However, once they are named and appropriated by the patient, they become part of the person's lifeworld. Since the focus of this study is pain, I shall have little to say about medical signs.

To call a feeling a symptom is already to interpret it, and there is no necessity that a particular feeling will be so interpreted. Radley (1994) pointed out that situational and social contexts play a role in the interpreting – and this can mean even noticing – a felt bodily sense as a symptom. In fact, "symptoms do not necessarily precede sickness; instead, being deemed to be sick is an important element in appearing symptomatic" (p. 71). A felt bodily change may not be taken as a symptom. If I have been digging in the garden and then feel pain in my knees, I likely will not say that the pain is a symptom of any illness. But if out of the blue my knees hurt, I might think that I have symptoms of arthritis. Pain belongs to multiple interpretative schemas. Sullivan (2001) argued that "pain experience is an important part of the 'form of life' adopted by any human group. . . . Human pain is defined more in terms of its relations than its inherent qualities" (p. 151). One inquiry (Palmer et al., 2000) concluded that an increase in reported back pain did not reflect a "greater incidence of severe back disease," but that "cultural changes have led to a greater awareness of more minor back symptoms and willingness to report them, and this cultural shift may also have rendered back pain more acceptable as a reason for absence attributed to sickness" (p. 1578). A related study (Buchbinder, Jolley, & Wyatt, 2001) described how a public health campaign to change popular beliefs about back pain correlated with a reduction of claims for back pain. The complex interplay between pain and culture indicates that culture plays intricate roles in the appearance, endurance, and handling of pain (Buchbinder, 2010; Encandela, 1993; Good, 1994; Lupton, 1994). If pain is to be understood, it is not as an objective presence but as constructed.

Another way of stating the thesis of the construction of pain is to say that pain always entails interpretation. If this is so, then Peirce's semiotics can prove to be beneficial to understanding pain, for semiotics centers on the study of interpretative activities. Signs are what one interprets, with what one interprets, and the meanings of what one interprets, according to Peirce. From this perspective, the medical distinction between (subjective) symptom and (objective) sign collapses: Semiotically speaking, both are signs.

Signs, symptoms, and Peirce's semiotics

But what is a sign? According to Peirce:

> A sign, or *representamen*, is something which stands to somebody for something in some respect or capacity. It addresses somebody, that is, creates in the mind of that person an equivalent sign, or perhaps a more developed sign. That sign which it creates I call the *interpretant* of the first sign. The sign stands for something, its *object*. It stands for that object, not in all respects, but in reference to a sort of idea, which I have sometimes called the *ground* of the representamen.
>
> *(Peirce, 1960, p. 2.228;*[2] *italics in the original)*

In other words:

1 A sign signifies: A sign is a something, and "everything can be a sign to an organism given the proper circumstances" (Bouissac, 1998, p. 738). Felt bodily states such as twinges and throbbings, a painless blotch on the skin, the result of a blood test, signify something. In Peirce's terms, they are representamens.
2 A sign is interpreted: Something is a sign if and only if it is interpreted. This characteristic distinguishes it from both a cause and an effect. The taking of something as a sign need not be an intellectual interpretation. Being frightened when seeing a dentist's drill is as much an interpretant of the sight of the drill as is the dentist's dispassionate professional grasp of the drill.
3 A sign points beyond itself: A sign represents an object in some respect. For example, a pain (as a representamen) represents the abdomen as hiding an inflamed appendix. The object represented need not exist, of course. A unicorn is an imaginary object, but an object nonetheless. A false positive on a medical test is a sign that in fact refers to a no-thing. Someone today saying *my heart hurts* probably refers, in part at least, to *heart* as understood anatomically, whereas a similar expression from the Renaissance could have indicated another conception of the heart. The object as represented by the sign is itself, then, a sign. Semiosis or meaning making occurs when someone interprets something as standing for or pointing to something else.

The key to the Peircean understanding is the interpretant that the sign "creates" or "determines." A sign is not a sign without its interpretant, which in turn becomes a sign and so determines interpretants in a potentially infinite series. Peirce emphasized the triadic relation (object–representamen–interpretant) of semiotics, which differs from a dyadic cause–effect relation. A sign only means something to the interpretant (a thought, action, or feeling, for example): "The meaning of every thought is established by a triadic relation, an *interpretation* of the thought as a *sign* of a determining *object*" (Hoopes, 1991, p. 7; italics in the original). The interpretant takes the sign (the representamen) as meaning its object. Esposito (1999) held that the interpretant influences how the object produces the representamen: As in a sentence, the final word determines what the first words in a sentence mean. A key point is that it is the action or feeling that interprets, not an interpreter (Dewey, 1946). This point helps bring together the phenomenology of embodiment with Peircean semiotics, insofar as a felt bodily sense can act as an interpretant.

Eco's (1984) analysis built upon the Peircean model by emphasizing that "substitution . . . is not the only necessary condition for a sign: the possibility of *interpretation* is necessary as well" (p. 43; italics in the original). For Eco, "every *interpretant* (either a sign or an expression or a sequence of expressions which translate a previous expression), besides translating the Immediate Object or the content of the sign, also increases our understanding of it" (p. 43; italics in the original) – that is, an act of interpretation in producing an interpretant produces understanding. An interpretant is *about* the object via the sign. The interpretant situates the object in an interpretive framework. Discourse is semiotic activity insofar as the representamens give an account (the interpretant) of something (the object) within a community of relevance.

Peirce (1960) differentiated signs in a number of ways, the most important being the relation of a sign or representamen to its object. There are three ways in which a sign can relate to its object, and so there are three types of signs: the icon, the index, and the symbol. An *icon* "is a sign which refers to the Object that it denotes merely by virtue of characters of its own" (p. 2.247). An X-ray film, an anatomical map, a metaphor, and an algebraic formula are examples of icons. Pain is iconic insofar as it is not an object of my perception but rather as who and what I am, prereflectively: "I *am* the feeling, I do not *have* it" (Baer, 1986, p. 145; italics in the original). An *index* "is a sign which refers to the Object by virtue of being really affected by that Object" (p. 2.248). Smoke is an index of fire; sudden hair loss is an index of chemotherapy; pain in a joint is an index of arthritis. A felt bodily sense taken as a medical symptom is thus an index. A *symbol* "is a sign which refers to the Object that it denotes by virtue of a law, usually an association of general ideas, which operates to cause the Symbol to be interpreted as referring to that Object" (p. 2.249). The word *heart* is a symbol, as is the figure ♥. Symbols are conventional. The anatomical map, while an icon of the body in one respect, is also symbolic and differs from other symbol systems for the body, such as that of traditional Chinese medicine. The symptom as symbol has a place in one's narrative of illness and healing. A person may go to a Western-style medical doctor and to a *curandera*, integrating (or not) the different explanatory models that interpret the symptom.

The same sign can have iconic, indexical, and symbolic aspects. For example, a painting done in Renaissance perspective is iconic in that in viewing it, one can discover relations to the objects represented that were not initially noticed. It is indexical in that it is a trace of paint on canvas, a clue to the influence of objects on the painter, and symbolic in that perspective is a tradition in painting for depicting people, places, and things.

Peirce also addressed relationships between a sign and its interpretant, which need not be a concept. This point is helpful in connecting signs with understanding pain as attunement, as disturbance or rupture. Peirce differentiated emotional, energetic, and logical interpretants (see Muller, 2000, for psychoanalytic examples of these three interpretants). An emotional interpretant "is a feeling" (Peirce, 1960, p. 5.475) produced by a sign. He used as an example the emotional thrill when hearing a stirring piece of music. Second, energetic interpretants involve effort, such as a soldier obeying an order or the strain of trying to understand something that someone says. Third, logical interpretants involve the future, in that they entail some degree of generalization and understanding of what "would be" (p. 5.482). For example, we interpret a felt bodily sense as a symptom by what we do about it next.

Since the object that the sign stands for and the interpretant of the sign are themselves signs, we can consider a symptom as occupying in turn any one of the three positions. As an *object*, the symptom is what I feel: pain and fluttering in the chest. As a *representamen*, the symptom means I have 6 months to live. As an *interpretant*, the symptom (e.g., palpitations) occurs when the physician says *The lab tests indicate that you have cancer.* In their turn, the palpitations mean to the physician that the patient is afraid, and so the physician adds an anti-anxiety drug to his prescription list to counter that object (the palpitations). This winding through the labyrinth of the sign is the process of constructing meaning.

Pain and semiotics

Where does it hurt? Pain, especially physical pain, is often considered a symptom signaling danger. Sullivan (1998) observed that pain cannot be understood only as private and incommunicable:

> How do we know how much we hurt? There may not be as much difference . . . between "how we know how much we ourselves hurt" and "how we know how much someone else hurts" as is generally assumed.
>
> *(p. 192)*

Pain is an interpretation, and self-knowledge, as Sullivan implied, is not much different than knowledge of others. Situational circumstances play a role in whether we say that we are in pain or not, whether we call it "pain" or "an ache" or something else, whether we classify the pain as physical, emotional, or moral. Isolation, anger, and sadness figure into how and what is interpreted as painful. That pain can often deceive, as in the pain that comes too late to warn of the danger lurking within, shows that pain is a sign, for Eco (1984) wrote that only signs can lie and that one can lie only with them. Moreover, the loose connection between physical pain and physiological lesions confirms pain as a sign: It is not simply an effect of some cause, but its presence points to *something*.

Pain as an attunement antedates distinctions between inside and outside, self and other, cognition and feeling. It is simultaneously *my* finding myself, my *finding* myself, and my finding *myself*. Therefore, we can say that there are painful and pained understandings of self and world. This restates what we found in the previous chapter: that pain is an intentional relationship between self and world, manifesting disturbances and ruptures in existence. A pain understanding articulates the world in distinctive ways. These remarks can, with the aid of Peirce's conception of the sign, deepen an understanding of how pain "means." For if pain is a sign, pain can occupy any position in the sign triad. It can be an object: "I feel pain *there*." It can be the representamen: Pain *means* danger. It can be the interpretant: A headache *flares* after I have been insulted. Whereas pain has been viewed as both an object and a representamen, here I will stress consideration of pain as an interpretant.

Pain as object

Where does it hurt? Pain's rich sensory qualities, its locations in the body, the redness or sore or bruise that identify it, all point to pain as the object. Emotional pains also have their locations, as we have seen. Pain is not pain if it is not felt. Indeed, all pain, including moral pain, resonates corporeally.

Pain as representamen

Pain can mean something. It can warn of disease, overexertion, grief, or guilt. Aldrich and Eccleston (2000) described worrisome pain, good pain, labor pains, heartaches, backaches, referred pain, and so on as ways that pain represents something. Even if it means nothing at all and is a nameless terror, the pain is lived as opening up the chasm of endless torment. The behavioral and psychosomatic approaches to pain considered pain as a sign in this sense. Pain is a type of communication, at times an address to others for care or love. Not rewarding pain behavior attempts to change the object of the pain: from sympathy, for example, to nothing. Pain thus means something to the person feeling it and, in its display, means something to others. One way that pain signifies – one that is sustained in a variety of cultural ways and embedded in the very etymology of the word *pain* – is that pain means punishment. Justice systems turn on the delivery of pain as a means of punishing illegal activity. Christie (1981/2007) demonstrated that criminal justice systems operate by inflicting pain, and the pain is intended to mean something in addition to punishment: In assigning greater and lesser penalties for different crimes, "pain delivery is here used as a moral declaration" (p. 35), thereby asserting a hierarchy of values. If I experience the pain of disease as punishment, although this "may seem inappropriate and even anti-therapeutic to the physician," it "may nonetheless preserve a sense of self-identity for the sufferer in the face of the impersonal rationality which bio-medicine may seek to impose" (Bendelow & Williams, 1995, p. 154). In one sense, cultures are the chief ways that pain comes to mean something. Theodicies, penal codes, and educational justifications of pain bear on pain as representamen. If pain is punishment for sin or the just desserts for bad choices, its significance is iconic: The pain participates in the reality it presents. Cultures, in particular religions, define symbolic meanings of pain.

Pain as interpretant

This aspect of pain as a sign is less familiar because pain is usually taken as *what* we feel rather than a *way* in which we feel. Olivier's (2007) philosophical phenomenology of pain converges with the idea that pain is an interpretant: "Pain is a mode of bodily perception. It denotes how I perceive – sense, feel and think – and thereby how I relate to my environment and to myself" (p. 48). By "bodily perception," he means the lived body – not the anatomical image of the body – so his statement could be modified to read that pain is a mode of embodied perceiving (sensing, feeling, thinking) that is grasped initially prereflectively. It is a way in which embodied subjectivity encounters and knows its world.

Here is an example of pain as interpretant. A young woman visits her physician, complaining of stomach pain. A medical examination reveals "nothing" and, in particular, a pregnancy test is negative. That last result announced, the pain recedes. The change in pain, its lessening, interprets the test result. It is not that she was feigning pain; it is that the lessened pain interpreted the sign (the test). Other common scenarios include headaches worsening after a patient is told they point to a tumor; "job dissatisfaction and unsatisfactory social relations in the workplace" (Morris, 1998, p. 119) predict back pain. A former student wrote to me and said *Whenever I get close to the campus, my stomach hurts.* The stomach pain discloses the sight of the campus as something to avoid. She cannot stomach the place, as we say.

The typical interpretation of such correlations is in dyadic terms: The pain is an effect produced by a stimulus. Without denying that indexical aspect of a sign, it is also the case that pain interprets the event as an act of the subject. Pain as interpretant helps us comprehend the oft-cited finding (Beecher, 1956; Wall, 1979) that there is no one-to-one correlation between tissue damage and pain. Consider the commonplace scene of a young child sprinting across a kitchen, tripping and hitting a knee on the floor. For a split second, the child's eye catches Mother's eye. What does she do? If she grimaces, the child bursts into tears, the knee filled with pain. If she reacts matter-of-factly, the child gets up and keeps on running. Here, the pain interprets the mother's look of anguish. Again, the diagnosis of cancer can be interpreted by the patient as a pain in a part of the body that theretofore was a curious presence or sore. The patient's pain interprets the diagnosis. A final example comes from Lafaille (1992): "Emotional or existential pain may be accompanied by physical pain, such as pain in the region of the heart, for example, after bereavement" (p. 187). Expressed in Peircean terms, the heart pain means the absence of the person who has died. Pain as interpretant can affect a person's lifeworld as such. Bendelow and Williams (1995) noted that "pain re-organises our lived space and time, our relations with others and with ourselves" (p. 148). More generally, pain changes things: Someone with severe back pain would see an automobile trip or a flight of stairs not as something that beckons but as a veritable instrument of torture. One reads the situation through the lens of pain, which "translates" the car or the stairs into the "language" of back pain. These examples show the interlinking of object, representamen, and interpretant in the semiotic triad of pain.

Stress and pain

We know about the pain of others by what they say and do. In listening to narratives in which pain figures prominently, consider the commonplace that stress causes pain and causes it to worsen and that stress reduction can alleviate pain (Shigaki, Glass, & Schopp, 2006; Westgaard, 1999). Rather than a critical analysis of stress (Jackson, 2013; Kugelmann, 1992), simply take it as part of our symbolic order of illness and health. This analysis will reinterpret what are typically presented as dyadic causal or correlative relationships into triadic relationships of signs.

The example returns to an interview I had with a man who had been injured at work whom I had discussed in Chapter 4. He stated that the causes of the accident were "our boss was pushing us, you know, I figure it was just my day to get hurt." Pain occurred as an object, a representamen, and an interpretant in the interview. What we primarily discussed, however, was not the pain per se but himself as a man – that is, as someone capable of doing anything, of being strong, and of being in control of his emotions. When he spoke of stress, it was primarily as it interpreted his current inability to do things (work, carry out garbage, pick up his child) because of the pain such activities caused. In this context, pain was a sign of his perhaps not being a man anymore. He understood manhood in terms of bringing home a paycheck and being "strong-minded" vis-à-vis authority figures and others who exploit signs of weakness. Pain was a representamen of his being a man. It was thus also a contested object for him, since he interpreted what he heard in the pain management program as meaning that the pain was "in his head," whereas he insisted it was in the "bulging discs" in his back, a consequence of his injury and of the injustice he suffered. Lack of trust in his doctors and his employer interpreted his pain. His continuing pain interpreted his conviction about the cause of his pain. The persistence of pain interpreted what he heard, as increases in pain interpreted his failed efforts to do things that he formerly could.

Stress was a term he used to indicate how he interpreted his inability to do the things that defined him as a man. In his terms, pain caused stress; semiotically, stress (the tension, the anxiety, etc.) interpreted pain as an object. More specifically, he said, because of stress, he "blows up and lashes out at his family" because he cannot do things as a result of his pain. The stress he felt (the representamen) referred to his back pain and resulted in rage (the interpretant). We can say that pain, as his way of finding himself (an interpretant) when he tried to be a man, was both a medical symptom and an object of his concern, especially of his wounded manhood.

Three comments are in order: First, this particular pain entailed an interpretive framework in which "being a man" has a specific cultural significance (Noone & Stephens, 2008). Second, as Peirce (1960) noted, every sign, in being related to its interpretants, has a rhetorical aspect: how "one sign gives birth to another, and especially one thought brings forth another" (p. 2.229). The man's narrative sought to persuade me, whom he identified with the psychologists in the hospital who were trying to convince him that the pain was in his head, that he was a man and that his pain was caused by damage in his back. What he said to me, then, interpreted his pain to me, and he did persuade me that the question of his self was at issue in his pain. Third, in addition to being symbolic, the pain was iconic, in that it was the weakness he so feared, and also indexical, an effect of his injury and the lack of reality he felt that the medical community afforded it.

From a Peircean perspective, social institutions in their organization and objectives determine triadic relationships. This man was struggling with the interpretations that he was being taught in the clinic. The clinic taught that stress was a big factor in the intensity of pain, a way of thinking that this patient understood as denying the reality of his pain. The program, in turn, was an interpretative framework carrying institutional authority that defined chronic pain. The program also sought to define the patient's self, in that it taught him that he was likely not to return to his preinjury pain-free status. Being in the program changed his pain, if in no other sense than that it altered the contexts in which he interpreted his pain. Pain took on new significance for him in the program, whether he accepted the interpretations or not.

Critical reflections

Peircean semiotics is a useful analytic for a critical approach to health. The triadic structure of the sign enables specification of how a symptom like pain is a mode of being in the world with others. It does so by indicating how pain is an object of concern, a sign of some object, and an interpretant, in which self and world are known or revealed. Pain can be taken up by others in more ways than one: as a cry for help, as a sign of deception, as an unconscious seeking of secondary gain, and so on. It can be presented in these ways as well. The precise form of pain includes the social networks within which it occurs. What a Peircean analytic contributes is a means to specify the pivots of discourse and other practices that are simultaneously private and public.

How people interpret pain will lead to its being classified as physical pain, emotional or psychological pain, social pain, or moral pain. The same object can be interpreted in more than one way as well. For example, chronic back pain could represent damage to the spine and express distress over long-term unemployment. As a sign, moreover, pain can communicate meanings to the self and others, such as a need for comfort or security or grief over loss.

Willig's (2000) call to study "*how* discourse may be implicated in subjectivity and *how* experience may be mediated by discourse" (p. 553; italics in the original) is precisely what this semiotic can accomplish. Speech says something (to me, to a generalized other) and affects something (speech is action, speech affects action). If something signifies, it has rhetorical effect; it produces an interpretant in the self and in the other. Thus, Peirce's semiotics provides another means to understand how discourse or any act accomplishes social action. In the previous example, the man contested the behavioral interpretive framework for pain, and he attempted unsuccessfully to substitute a biomedical one, grounding his complaint as well in a cultural tradition of masculinity, self-reliance, and stoicism. His complaint interpreted the meaning of the hospital's program, as did his abrupt departure from it. Pain had no merely private or inner existence; it circulated throughout the social and semiotic web that not only defined it and its bearers but also alleviated or aggravated it. This last point is important: It is not only the interpretation of pain that is at stake; pain itself is at stake. Increases and decreases in pain occur within a social nexus.

Peircean semiotics enables us to focus on the actual significance of interpretative schemas in specific pain performances. Knowledge claims circulate within power networks, having different effects depending on who says what when to whom. In the previous example, the man used a biomedical conception of pain to counter a pain medicine understanding (Baszanger, 1998) of chronic pain: It was the bulging disks, it was the accident – and not the stress – that caused the pain. Essential to the pain management program was an interpretive framework emphasizing nonbiomedical contributions to the persistence of pain. Therefore, in the interpretive conflict, the patient used the biomedical model without persuasive authority to legitimize his suffering in the face of what he at times perceived to be a delegitimizing counterinterpretation in terms of stress and pain behavior. In addition, he called upon cultural ideals to legitimize his interpretations of his suffering.

The semiotic approach shows the interweaving of culturally defined conceptions of the self (as a man, as self-controlled) with ways of interpreting pain. The processes of sign making indicate that interpretative frameworks are not simply impositions on people but that people actively take them up, express, interpret, and apply them to new ends. The analysis shows the intimate tie between pain and identity. Peirce (1960) alluded to this intimacy, stating that "man is a sign" (p. 5.310). Especially when intractable, pain, as a way of being in a situation, places who I thought I was into question. If only it could simply be an object that I have to tolerate. But pain, in addition, is my answer, my grasp, my understanding of the situation I find myself in. Pain is an unwelcome mode of being, one that I reject, and in my rejecting, I interpret the painfulness of pain. My very being, my existing, is repulsive to me in pain. How could it not raise the question of identity? Critical approaches to health need to address the context-specific constitution of pain, illness, healing, and health, as well as reckon with the larger social, cultural, and historical frameworks within which human action and experience take place. The triadic structure of the sign, especially conceived in a hermeneutic approach, furthers both theory and research options. For by considering the sign, we locate our studies not at the entities that are the residues, as it were, of semiotic action, but at the site where these entities – subject and object, mind and body, sickness and health – are constituted. Pain occurs in a complex semiotic web, takes place structurally as a situation, and exists through the agents who embody it in a variety of ways. Pain may be, to some extent, a private phenomenon, but it is, at the same time, a medium within which we share a common life.

Notes

1 This chapter is a revision of a 2003 article of mine, "Pain as Symptom, Pain as Sign." *Health: An Interdisciplinary Journal for the Social Study of Health, Illness and Medicine, 7*, 29–50.

2 The *Collected Papers* are organized by volume and paragraph number. This signifies Volume 2, paragraph 228.

References

Aldrich, S., & Eccleston, C. (2000). Making sense of everyday pain. *Social Science & Medicine, 50*, 1631–1641.

Baer, E. (1986). The medical symptom. In J. Deely, B. Williams, & F. E. Kruse (Eds.), *Frontiers in semiotics* (pp. 140–152). Bloomington: Indiana University Press.

Baszanger, I. (1998). *Inventing pain medicine: From the laboratory to the clinic.* New Brunswick, NJ: Rutgers University Press.

Beecher, H. K. (1956). Relationship of significance of wound to pain experienced. *Journal of the American Medical Association, 161*(17), 1609–1613. http://dx.doi.org/10.1001/jama.1956.02970170005002

Bendelow, G. A., & Williams, S. J. (1995). Transcending the dualisms: Towards a sociology of pain. *Sociology of Health and Illness, 17*, 139–165.

Bouissac, P. (1998). Converging parallels: Semiotics and psychology in evolutionary perspective. *Theory & Psychology, 8*, 731–753.

Buchbinder, M. (2010). Giving an account of one's pain in the anthropological interview. *Culture, Medicine and Psychiatry, 34*, 108–131. http://dx.doi.org/10.1007/s11013-009-9162-2

Buchbinder, R., Jolley, D., & Wyatt, M. (2001). Population based intervention to change back pain beliefs and disability: Three part evaluation. *BMJ, 322*, 1516–1520.

Christie, N. (2007). *Limits to pain: The role of punishment in penal policy.* Eugene, OR: Wipf & Stock. (Original work published 1981)

Dewey, J. (1946). Peirce's theory of linguistic signs, thought, and meaning. *Journal of Philosophy, 43*, 85–95.

Eco, U. (1984). *Semiotics and the philosophy of language.* Bloomington: Indiana University Press.

Encandela, J. A. (1993). Social science and the study of pain since Zborowski: A need for a new agenda. *Social Science & Medicine, 36*, 783–791.

Esposito, J. L. (1999). Peirce's theory of semiosis: Toward a logic of mutual affection. Cyber Semiotic Institute. Retrieved from www.chass.utoronto.ca/epc/srb/cyber/esp6.html

Good, B. (1994). *Medicine, rationality and experience: An anthropological perspective.* Cambridge, England: Cambridge University Press.

Hoopes, J. (1991). Introduction. In J. Hoopes (Ed.), *Peirce on signs: Writings on semiotics by Charles Sanders Peirce* (pp. 1–13). Chapel Hill: University of North Carolina Press.

Jackson, M. (2013). *The age of stress: Science and the search for stability.* Oxford, England: Oxford University Press.

Kugelmann, R. (1992). *Stress: The nature and history of engineered grief.* Westport, CT: Praeger.

Lafaille, R. (1992). Pain: A symptom of disintegrated life. *WHO Regional Publications, European Series, 44*, 182–184.

Lupton, D. (1994). *Medicine as culture: Illness, disease and the body in Western societies.* London, England: Sage.

Morris, D. (1998). *Illness and culture in the postmodern age.* Berkeley: University of California Press.

Müller, J. (2000). Hierarchical models in semiotics and psychoanalysis. In J. Müller & J. Brent (Eds.), *Peirce, semiotics, and psychoanalysis* (pp. 49–67). Baltimore, MD: Johns Hopkins University Press.

Noone, J. H., & Stephens, C. (2008). Men, masculine identities, and health care utilisation. *Sociology of Health & Illness, 30*, 711–725. http://dx.doi.org/10.1111/j.1467-9566.2008.01095.x

Olivier, A. (2007). *Being in pain.* Frankfurt, Germany: Lang.

Palmer, K. T., Walsh, K., Bendall, H., Cooper, C., & Coggon, D. (2000). Back pain in Britain: Comparison of two prevalence surveys at an interval of 10 years. *BMJ, 320*, 1577–1578.

Peirce, C. S. (1960). *Collected papers.* Cambridge, MA: Harvard University Press.

Radley, A. (1994). *Making sense of illness: The social psychology of health and disease.* London, England: Sage.

Shigaki, C. L., Glass, B., & Schopp, L. H. (2006). Mindfulness-based stress reduction in medical settings. *Journal of Clinical Psychology in Medical Settings, 13*, 209–216. http://dx.doi.org/10.1007/s10880-006-9033-8

Sullivan, M. D. (1998). Perspectives on pain and suffering. *Advances in Mind–Body Medicine, 14*, 167–203.

Sullivan, M. D. (2001). Finding pain between minds and bodies. *Clinical Journal of Pain, 17*, 146–156.

Wall, P. D. (1979). On the relation of injury to pain. *Pain, 6*, 253–264.

Westgaard, R. H. (1999). Effects of physical and mental stressors on muscle pain. *Scandinavian Journal of Work, Environment and Health, 25*, 19–24.

Willig, C. (2000). A discourse-dynamic approach to the study of subjectivity in health. *Theory & Psychology, 10*, 547–570.

8

MORAL PAIN AND KNOWLEDGE

To conclude, we continue probing pain as an interpretant – that is, as an *active*–passive performance. Pain may not always have a purpose or a meaning, but it does place us in a precarious situation, where we are exposed and, leaning into the brink, we find disclosed something of ourselves and our worlds. Thus far, we have seen that pain can signify different dimensions of living simultaneously, corporeally, psychologically, emotionally, and morally. Now we look explicitly at moral pain, extending the category of pain beyond the bounds of the discipline of psychology.

We have already encountered moral aspects of pain. The plaints and complaints of chronic pain sufferers raised the question of the justice of their situations. One of the women lamented, as we saw in Chapter 4:

> And I mean, I was like, God, I hope you're never on the end of the rope similar to yours because "what goes around comes around." And one of these days, somebody's going to do you the same way that you're doing your own employees.

She felt her injury as violating the natural justice of the world, an imbalance that she felt in her ongoing pain. It is worth noting that the etymology of *injury* is a word meaning *unjust* and that the earliest usage of *pain* signified punishment as well as bodily and mental suffering. We construct pain, and some of the material we use in doing so concerns justice, balance, fairness, good, and evil. In the previous chapter was another example – that of the young man whose pain threatened his sense of masculinity. This man's pain had several simultaneous significations. His pain was physical, a result of the injury he sustained; his pain was emotional, a result of the limitations it imposed on his life; his pain was moral, in that he felt it as a result of injustice in the workplace, compounded by the injustice, as he saw it, of not being taken seriously in the pain management program. His pain meant all of this at the same time.

Moral pain has entered psychological discourse in recent years in the context of the wounds of war. Therefore, we will look at moral pain in the context of warfare and at the phenomenon of "moral injury" suffered by soldiers in recent wars. Such wounds result from experiences with evil. Moral pain exposes individuals to knowledge that can overcome them, for good or for ill.

Moral pain

Moral pain was a type of pain recognized in the generation of Henry Rutgers Marshall, who argued against reducing pain to an effect of the stimulation of peripheral nerves. In the nineteenth century, the existence of moral pain appears to have been taken for granted. In *Utilitarianism*, John Stuart Mill (1863) argued that pleasures are various and not confined to "those of which swine are capable" (p. 10). A hierarchy of pleasures exists, such that "the pleasures of the intellect, of the feelings and imagination, and of the moral sentiments" have "a much higher value as pleasures than to those of mere sensation" (p. 11). In brief, there are "*kinds* of pleasures" (p. 11; italics in the original). As with pleasures, so with pains. He discussed "the positive evils of life, the great sources of physical and mental suffering – such as indigence, disease, and the unkindness, worthlessness, or premature loss of objects of affection" (p. 21). In a letter to Auguste Comte in 1843, Mill wrote how "sad I felt upon learning how the inveterate distaste you feel in a position, so little suited to your taste, has now been compounded by moral pain" (Haac, 1995, p. 83). Mill was referring to marital difficulties that Comte was facing: His wife of 17 years had left him, and he felt betrayed. "Moral pain" was significant in both registers – the emotional and the ethical.

A medical account of moral pain described it as "the biting of teeth which, once fleshed in sin, now tear the heart of the evil-doer" ("Remorse in Melancholia," 1906, p. 1319). This article discussed "moral pain" as "a realization of the shortcomings of some actual conduct . . . founded on logical concepts of good and evil" (p. 1319). The article also claimed that the physiological concomitants of melancholia could produce feelings that the patient interpreted as the moral pain of guilt.

Whatever the precise denotation, moral pain referred to the ethical realm. Its reality and its ethical import were stoutly defended: "Moral pain is just as real as physical pain, and if a wife is entitled to be protected against being beaten, she is also entitled, so far as liberty is concerned, to be protected against moral suffering" (Cecil, 1910, p. 20). In this assertion by the British politician and author Hugh Cecil, we see that the meaning of pain included meanings that were abandoned with the rise of the sensation theory. To illustrate the rejection of the broader notion of pain after the sensation theory became the received view, consider this pronouncement by the experimental psychologist Adolf Wohlgemuth (1917), for whom "pain is a sensation":

> Pain, in the proper psychological sense of the term, must not be confounded with what is called pain in the ordinary parlance and which is distinguished

> as "physical or bodily pain" and "mental or moral pain." . . . Mental or moral pain . . . has nothing whatever to do with pain, being merely the unpleasant affective content of a mental experience.
>
> *(p. 462)*

This way of constructing experience prevailed for decades.

In the mid-twentieth century, Buytendijk (1962) made a case for moral pain:

> Despite the essential differences between the "vital" and ethical spheres, both in regard to origin and relationship to self, a distinct ethical *life* exists. . . . In every sphere of "vital," aesthetic, and ethical values a man can be happy and he can be painfully afflicted and suffer.
>
> *(p. 136; italics in the original)*

To be sure, one's "personal participation in the ethical sphere" (p. 136) can vary, and some achieve immunity against ethical norms. In the ethical sphere of living, a wrong is painful; it wounds a person, either directly, by suffering the wrong, or indirectly, by witnessing a wrong suffered by another. Extending the analogy between physical and moral wounds, Buytendijk observed: "What we call the 'vital' should be regarded as a particular manifestation of an ethical order rather than as a specific instance of conformity to the laws governing the 'vital' sphere" (p. 137). This phenomenological analysis conforms to what we have found about pain as an attunement, in which physiological (vital) life belongs to the living of a person. Buytendijk's account also conforms to a semiotic reading of pain, in that pain is always an interpretation. A physical wound may resonate not only in the vital sphere but also in the emotional and moral spheres of living.

Buytendijk's assertions have received support from more recent research. DeWall and Baumeister (2006) found that "socially excluded participants consistently showed both decreased sensitivity and increased tolerance to physical pain" (p. 11). That is, social pain affected the feeling of corporeal pain, indicating that pain resonates into various spheres of living. Extending this line of thinking, Sivanathan and Zhong (2011) observed that "physical pain helps people withstand their social suffering, and in turn can reduce their motivation to help those in need" (p. 84). In other words, physical pain substituted for the moral pain that might lead to charitable acts. Moral pain is aptly called pain.

The more serious the pain, whether corporeal or psychological, the more it has moral implications. This formulation is ambiguous, and Crossley (2000) warned against remoralizing pain and illness, such that they are seen as punishment for a life ill led. Avoiding the presumption of blaming those in pain for their pain, we see that pain can signify the moral dimension of life in two ways: in terms of the ethical challenges it poses for those who would relieve pain and in terms of the suffering of evil by the ones in pain. It is the second of these two senses that shall occupy us here.

Moral pain and warfare

The category of moral pain has returned to American psychology in the wake of recent wars, starting with the war in Vietnam. An early reference to the moral pain suffered by veterans came from Peter Marin. Marin (1981) differentiated moral pain from the then-emerging category of "stress," based on an understanding that the language of psychology and the therapeutic approach were inadequate for the "moral distress" (p. 68) of these veterans. He described types of moral pain, the first being the pain of guilt, "a person's reaction to past actions he or she finds inexcusable or inexplicable" (p. 77). Second is "the way we internalize and experience as our own the disorder, suffering, and brutality around us," what he called "the world's pain" (p. 79). This pain can arise from "a pervasive sense of suffering, injustice, and evil" (p. 79). Finally, there is the pain of suffering "when we cannot act out in the world our response to the suffering we have seen in it" (p. 79). This inability concerns the desire to rectify the wrongs seen or committed. For Marin, this meant acting "in history" (p. 80), not simple behavior. This "imprisonment" (p. 80) returns us to the phenomenological sense that the place of pain is a threshold that can neither be dwelled in or passed across.

The psychiatrist Jonathan Shay saw continuity between the moral pain suffered by today's veterans and those of Achilles in the *Iliad*. Shay (1991) identified leadership's betrayal of soldiers as a most significant moral injury, comparing it to that felt by Achilles when his commander, Agamemnon, dishonored him, a wound initiating the action of the *Iliad*. Betrayal is a possibility because, as Shay (1994) argued, "an army is a moral construction" (p. 5). In addition to betrayal, Litz et al. (2009) found other events producing moral injury, including the killing of civilians, either deliberately or accidentally; seeing human remains; committing atrocities; and the death of a friend. This is a partial listing. They define moral injury as "perpetuating, failing to prevent, bearing witness to, or learning about acts that transgress deeply held moral beliefs and expectations" (p. 700).

It is important to consider the moral dimension of war, and even if war is rarely good, the fact that we recognize its evil locates it in the moral sphere of life. In addition to the obvious evil of slaughter and destruction, however, is the "moral construction" of the military (Shay, 1994). Military organization, authority, and individual expectations and loyalties, among other things, combine to "form a moral world that most of the participants most of the time regard as legitimate, 'natural,' and personally binding" (p. 6). Shay depicts what follows when a soldier is betrayed by leadership, as was Achilles. The betrayal, the hypocrisy, and the lies violate "what's right" and inflict moral injury. The suffering of that injury is moral pain. Other moral injuries arise from a soldier's experience of having committed or witnessed evil acts. Compounding this violence is "self-handicapping and self-harm, which are inflicted as punishment for moral transgression" (Jinkerson, 2014, p. 16). In this way, psychological and physical pains supplement, and perhaps attempt to alleviate, moral pain.

In each of these situations, pain from a type of wound or injury interpreted the situation as wrong, the world as ruptured. Moral pain may be the most significant way in which human beings recognize the disorder we call evil. Along this line, Warren Kinghorn (2012) warned against treating moral injuries as simply problems in terms of "the means-ends logic of technical rationality" (p. 65). Why? Because despite the "family resemblance" between "psychological and moral injuries" and "flesh-and-blood injuries" (p. 64), they differ in a significant way, making their treatment different as well. Kinghorn especially argued against medicalizing moral injury:

> Visible wounds to the body, however they might affect the experiencing self, can be formally identified without specific consideration of the soldier's response to them . . . the wound can be considered apart from, and in some sense prior to, its effect on the experiencing self. In the case of psychological and moral injury, on the other hand, the wound is known only through the soldier's psychological and moral response to the experience of combat; epistemologically, it *is* that response.
>
> *(p. 64; italics in the original)*

This statement needs qualification, since tissue damage and pain regularly involve not only a personal response to them but also their construction, as we have seen with chronic pain. Nevertheless, Kinghorn's distinction recalls that of Buytendijk, for whom pain can strike the individual in the different spheres of living, from the vital to the moral. A bodily wound and a moral wound afflict the possibility for the flourishing of the person in different ways, even granting the ways they overlap. A qualitative study (Currier, McCormick, & Drescher, 2015) found (among the psychological aspects of events that were morally injurious) hopelessness, pleasure in aggressive acts, emotional numbness, helplessness, desire for revenge, changed sense of self, and grief (p. 110). They found organizational, environmental, and cultural circumstances figuring into the production of moral injuries. The construction of moral pain entails a great variety of ruptures and disturbances in existence. In war, they tend to be serious.

Moral pain and injustice

Moral pain occurs in other circumstances as well. One form of evil is racism, and it too produces moral pain in those subject to it and in those who perpetrate it. Ralph Ellison (1964) wrote of the way that William Faulkner portrayed African Americans in his novels. Some characters embodied a "malignant stereotype" and a "benign stereotype" in an unintegrated way:

> The dual function of this dissociation seems to be that of avoiding moral pain and thus to justify the South's racial code. But since such a social order harms whites no less than blacks, the sensitive Southerner, the artist, is apt to feel its effects acutely – within the deepest levels of his personality.
>
> *(p. 42)*

Part of Ellison's point was that one ought to feel moral pain, especially when one's way of life contributes to and even benefits from the injustices. Laurence M. Thomas (1998) described the moral pain inflicted on individuals in "diminished social categories," which include "gender, ethnicity, and race" (p. 364). Diminished social category persons are constructed in intergroup relations: "In an oppressive society, the victims of oppression . . . are constituted . . . so as not to see themselves as full and equal members of society" (p. 365). Members of privileged groups can contribute to this constitution without intentionally meaning to do so: "Except for the blatant bigot or sexist, participating in the downward social constitution of another rarely has any special phenomenological feel to it" (p. 366). As a result, becoming aware of the moral pain suffered by such individuals may be difficult for the nondownwardly constituted to grasp. Moral pain may look like shame or hostility, for example. As with chronic pain, moral pain can be invisible to others.

Listening to the morally pained

As we have seen, those in chronic pain are hurting and yet sometimes not believed. This dismissal of their experience compounds their corporeal pain with moral pain, the pain of injustice. It is all too often invisible. Ellison's novel *Invisible Man* (1952) is the story of another type of invisibility – that of a black man in a racist society. The basic metaphor is easy to determine: The narrator, Ellison's Underground Man, is not seen as who he is, not seen as an individual person, but as a type, less than fully human. While the discrimination that those in chronic pain face differs from racial discrimination, there is at least one point of contact: the invisibility of the person who suffers from the moral pain of injustice.

Thomas's (1998) provocative essay "Moral Deference" has insights that the critical approach to pain needs to reckon with. He inquired into the "appropriate and inappropriate responses to the moral pain of another" (p. 362) – particularly to the moral pain suffered by individuals subject to racism and other forms of discrimination. There is no symmetry between the experiences of those subject to racism and those who are not subject to it. It would be presumptuous for those with privileged social status to assume that they can understand the moral pain of people who are the objects of racism. This lack of understanding happens "because the individual is speaking from a vantage point to which someone not belonging to his diminished social category group does not have access" (p. 374). Moral deference, then, is "the act of listening involved in bearing witness to another's moral pain, but without bearing witness to it" (p. 377). Such listening can give one "a new set of sensibilities" (p. 377) – in particular, "to engage in moral deference is to allow oneself to become affected in a direct interpersonal way by the injustices of this world" (p. 378).

These considerations recall the ways in which the individuals with chronic pain complained about the injustices of their condition. They, too, cried out for justice and apology. Listening to them, as in listening to those who suffer moral pain, requires the perspective that Levinas (1969) addressed: That the other person – in particular "the stranger, the widow, and the orphan" (p. 77) to use his examples – speak to me from beyond my own particular world and that in a fundamental way, I cannot comprehend them. The Other exceeds my grasp. As a result, I cannot grasp the pain of another, but I can listen and work to alleviate it.

Moral pain reveals evil

Carlo Maggini (2005) identified moral pain as a state "experienced in response to negative life events and turns of fate" (p. 53), aligning it with something that used to be called *melancholy*. Melancholy, in this sense, is not an illness but a reasoned perspective on human events. Melancholy remains aware that " 'even in the midst of laughing there is sorrow,' . . . even in the midst of all our feasting and jollity . . . there is grief and discontent" (Burton, 1883, pp. 93–94). Melancholy, as a kind of attunement in Heidegger's sense, is the disposition capable of beginning to grasp moral pain.

It is beyond the scope of this consideration of moral pain to address its alleviation. We only are considering what moral pain reveals about the world. For many soldiers, the experience of moral pain shatters preconceptions that "the world is benevolent, the world is meaningful, and the self is worthy" (Litz et al., 2009, p. 698). Moral pain entails terrible semiotic activity. The flare of such pain has many occasions, as the literature on it demonstrates. Sticking with Shay's (2014) conception of it, "where leadership malpractice inflicts moral injury, the body codes it as physical attack, mobilizes for danger and counterattack" (p. 185). In other words, leadership malpractice, experienced as such by the soldier, reveals the world to be otherwise than he or she thought. Moral injury is an end of innocence. The pain of such a wound is shadow knowledge, felt with the aversion or repulsion that characterizes the passive activity of pain. The person perceives the actual presence of evil, and this perceiving is the wounding. Shay observed that moral injury destroyed trust; then, a person expected "harm, exploitation, and humiliation" (2014, p. 188). Not only does trust in others suffer in such wounding; part of the pain is loss of trust in oneself.

The wound of moral pain is not necessarily tissue damage to the body, although it may be. What is significant, as Kinghorn (2012) indicates, is that "the conflicts, dissonances, and moral emotions characteristic of moral injury are those of a moral agent, an acting person" (p. 62). Because moral pain implies an experiencing moral agent, the pain is an interpretant perceiving the wound as meaning that evil has happened. With moral pain, we return to the images given in the first pages of this book: Once upon a time, there was no pain. In the cosmological accounts of the Book of Genesis and Greek myth, pain entered the world when evil was unleashed. If physical pains deal with physical evils (sharp knives in the flesh, for example), moral pains deal with deeper strata of disorder, violence, and degradation.

Just as the category of moral pain revives an older notion, so the response to moral pain draws upon older traditions as well. Bernard Verkamp (1993) described religious rituals that flourished in the early medieval period, when returning warriors regularly partook in penitential rites to cleanse them of the sin of partaking in the violence of war, even if the war had been deemed just. Although "the necessity of the campaigns of which they were a part" (Kinghorn, 2012, p. 69) was affirmed, with the war being the "lesser of two evils," the rites acknowledged it as still evil. What needs healing in moral pain is more than medicine and psychology, or any critical approach to health, can manage. Pain knows evil in this, the widest sphere of human existence. Evil is not managed.

Critical reflections

This excursion into moral pain was designed to demonstrate that pain is an interpretant, a way of actively engaging with the world – whether we want to or not. With these considerations, our examination of ways in which we construct pain in the contemporary world is at an end. The shape of the narrative has been like an hourglass. A broad view of pain as a feeling, as a quality of consciousness, gave way to a narrow perspective rooted in the anatomical image of the body and resulting in "real pain." This constricted construction is still with us, but it has been challenged in various ways. The intractability of some pains, called *chronic*, called for new constructions that did not fit the mold of brief and acute pain. With the acknowledgment of the complexities of pain, we widened the scope again, seeing how psychological pain is indeed pain. An excursion through phenomenological accounts of pain showed that pain entails a world that is formed along with an embodied subject. Pain is an affliction of personal existence in a variety of ways. It is constructed in a semiotic process, signifying affliction. Its widest extent is that of the moral sphere of life. Pain takes place as an impossible passive activity in the face of a wound to existence. It attunes us to the flaws and disturbances, the gaps and fissures, in our lives. It teaches us about evil.

Pain remains volatile, a potent symbol of disorder in the cosmos. However, it should teach one that when taking a critical approach to health, that when entering into dialogue and relationship with those in pain, we tread on sacred ground. Pain is indeed constructed – made and done – by individuals and by cultures. It is not, however, simply constructed. It remains, like eros, most uncultivated, unconstructed, wild, formless, intimate, and remote.

References

Burton, R. (1883). *The anatomy of melancholy.* Philadelphia, PA: Claxton.

Buytendijk, F.J.J. (1962). *Pain: Its modes and functions* (E. O'Shiel, Trans.). Chicago, IL: University of Chicago Press.

Cecil, H. (1910). *Liberty and authority.* London, England: Arnold.

Crossley, M. L. (2000). *Rethinking health psychology.* Philadelphia, PA: Open University Press.

Currier, J. M., McCormick, W., & Drescher, K. D. (2015). How do morally injurious events occur? A qualitative analysis of perspectives of veterans with PTSD. *Traumatology, 21*(2), 106–116. http://dx.doi.org/10.1037/trm0000027

DeWall, C. N., & Baumeister, R. F. (2006). Alone but feeling no pain: Effects of social exclusion on physical pain tolerance and pain threshold, affective forecasting, and interpersonal empathy. *Journal of Personality and Social Psychology, 91*(1), 1–15. http://dx.doi.org/10.1037/0022-3514.91.1.1

Ellison, R. (1952). *Invisible man.* New York, NY: Random House.

Ellison, R. (1964). *Shadow and act.* New York, NY: Random House.

Haac, O. A. (1995). *The correspondence of John Stuart Mill and Auguste Comte* (O. A. Haac, Ed. & Trans.). New Brunswick, NJ: Transaction.

Jinkerson, J. (2014). Moral injury as a new normal in the modern wars. *The Military Psychologist, 29*(3), 16–18.

Kinghorn, W. (2012). Combat trauma and moral fragmentation: A theological account of moral injury. *Journal of the Society of Christian Ethics, 32*, 57–74.

Levinas, E. (1969). *Totality and infinity* (A. Lingis, Trans.). Pittsburgh, PA: Duquesne University Press.

Litz, B. T., Stein, N., Delaney, E., Lebowitz, L., Nash, W. P., Silva, C., & Maguen, S. (2009). Moral injury and moral repair in war veterans: A preliminary model and intervention strategy. *Clinical Psychology Review, 29*, 695–706. http://dx.doi.org/10.1016/j.cpr.2009.07.003

Maggini, C. (2005). Moral pain and senility. *Acta Biomedica, 76*, 53–59.

Marin, P. (1981). Living in moral pain. *Psychology Today, 15*(11), 68–80.

Mill, J. S. (1863). *Utilitarianism.* London, England: Parker, Son and Bourn.

Remorse in melancholia. (1906). *British Medical Journal, 2*(2393), 1319–1320.

Shay, J. (1991). Learning about combat stress from Homer's *Iliad*. *Journal of Traumatic Stress, 4*, 561–579. http://dx.doi.org/10.1002/jts.2490040409

Shay, J. (1994). *Achilles in Vietnam: Combat trauma and the undoing of character.* New York, NY: Scribner.

Shay, J. (2014). Moral injury. *Psychoanalytic Psychology, 31*, 182–191.

Sivanathan, N., & Zhong, C.-B. (2011). Hurting the body . . . and the soul: Physical pain can mitigate moral pain. In R. Ahluwalia, T. L. Chartrand, & R. K. Ratner (Eds.), *NA – Advances in consumer research* (Vol. 39, p. 84). Duluth, MN: Association for Consumer Research.

Thomas, L. M. (1998). Moral deference. In C. Willet (Ed.), *Theorizing multiculturalism* (pp. 359–381). Malden, MA: Blackwell.

Verkamp, B. J. (1993). *The moral treatment of returning warriors in early medieval and modern times.* Scranton, PA: University of Scranton Press.

Wohlgemuth, A. (1917). The feelings and their neural correlate, with an examination of the nature of pain. *British Journal of Psychology, 8*, 423–476. http://dx.doi.org/10.1111/j.2044-8295.1917.tb00141.x

INDEX

9781138841208